My Broken Vagina

One Woman's Quest to Fix Her Sex Life, and Yours

FRAN BUSHE

First published in Great Britain in 2021 by Hodder Studio
An Hachette UK company

1

A CIP catalogue record for this title is available from the British Library

Hardback ISBN 9781529347647
Trade Paperback ISBN 9781529347654
eBook ISBN 9781529347661

Typeset in Bembo by Hewer Text UK Ltd, Edinburgh
Printed and bound in Great Britain by Clays Ltd, Elcograf S.p.A.

Hodder & Stoughton policy is to use papers that are natural, renewable
and recyclable products and made from wood grown in sustainable forests.
The logging and manufacturing processes are expected to conform
to the environmental regulations of the country of origin.

Hodder & Stoughton Ltd
Carmelite House
50 Victoria Embankment
London EC4Y 0DZ

www.hodder-studio.com

Contents

For 16-year-old Fran, your hair will always be frizzy at the back, but I promise you sex will get better

A Note from a Weary Author

I hear you're writing a book about sex Fran.
3.00 a.m.

Hi, ex-boyfriend from the past.
8.32 a.m.

We've had sex.
8.37 a.m.

Yep.
9.00 a.m.

So, the book is about me?
9.01 a.m.

. . . No.
9.30 a.m.

But we've had sex.
9.32 a.m.

. . . Yep?
9.35 a.m.

So I'm the main character!?
9.37 a.m.

No.
9.45 a.m.

But the storyline is about me?
9.47 a.m.

You aren't in my book.
[Unimpressed smiley face]
9.57 a.m.

[Thinking smiley face]
WHY NOT?!!!
Put me in the book.
I think my skills should be immortalised in the literary canon!
10.00 a.m.

[Unimpressed smiley face]
11.00 a.m.

I mean make me anonymous, but say like . . . the cool one.
With a beard. That works in the Arts.
11.03 a.m.

That actually doesn't whittle you guys down.
At all.
1.04 p.m.

Let's meet. I can give you anecdotes
OR
be your editor
(I've written 3 best man speeches
now so am great at writing).
[smiley face]
10.54 p.m.

OR give you a little reminder of my skills . . .
[aubergine emoji] [winking smiley]
[acrobat emoji]
11.00 p.m.

U up Fran?
11.10 p.m.

Fran? U up?
12.05 a.m.

Fran?
2.34 a.m.

When I started speaking publicly about sex, nearly all of my past lovers got in touch. Long-term relationships, two-date Bumble swipes, anyone who had ever been remotely near my vagina.

Past lovers, this book is not about you. It is not a kiss and tell. It is not a tour de foreskin.

This book is about me and about sex. It is indisputable that a lot, in fact the majority of the sex I've had involved another human person, but this story is mine. It has been all about you for too, too, too long.

Ok, that is more than enough space to devote to you.

Now it is time for me.

Introduction

My name is Fran, I'm a writer and I have a vagina.

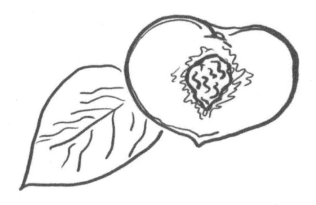

Let me try again . . . a vagina!

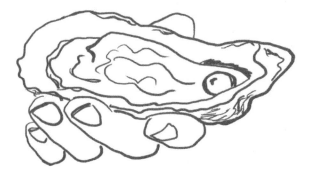

How about a vulva?

IMAGE NOT AVAILABLE

Right. Yes. I see.

We are used to seeing vulvas and vaginas visually represented as fresh fruits, exotic flowers, glistening shellfish or a hidden watering hole in a fertile mountain glade. So zesty, so fresh, so censored! For a really long time, I thought my vagina was broken. If mine was to star in an advert, it wouldn't have been a dewy orchid or a plump papaya. It would have been a drooping tulip or an angry-looking cuttlefish living in an algae-covered pond.

The trouble with representing genitalia as sea conches and mangoes is that it means the only vulva most heterosexual people with vaginas see is their own. Even this isn't guaranteed (a mirror and privacy and courage and awkward angles are often required for this feat). Someone looking through anatomy books is unlikely to find something that resembles their own genitalia, among scientifically symmetrical labia and neatly groomed mons pubis, sandwiched neatly, nearly always, between pale white slender legs. I didn't speak about or look at mine for a really long time. I mostly just imagined an 'out of order' sign dangling over my pants.

So here goes. Here is mine.

Ok, so I really wanted to draw my own vulva here, but I lost my nerve, mostly because in my head there was a horrified voice going 'Oh Fran, you put your vulva in your book?! How will you get an eligible husband now? Cover your vulva with a lace-trim bonnet immediately and get thee on a bicycle (notoriously uncomfortable for vulvas) in an eternal spin class of shame!' Plus, we barely know each other right now. Maybe once we've got more acquainted.

Though I didn't want to put my vulva in the opening pages of this book, I absolutely did have a go drawing it, and you can too! If you want. Or describe it. Or tear out this page to make an elaborate origami labia minora and majora. But also, no pressure.

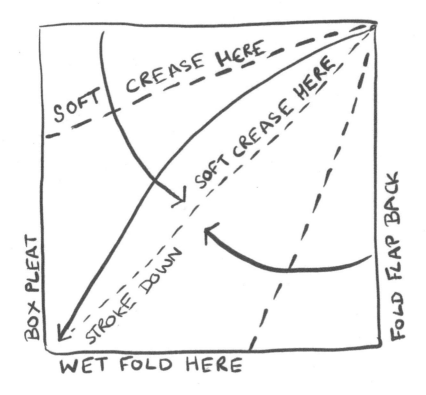

Your vulva is yours. I'm not suggesting that in reading this book you run out and immediately present your vulva to your CEO, mother-in-law or Uber driver (that might not be good for your rating). Some revolutions are loud and fierce, some are as simple as reading a book or fetching your hand mirror. What I would like is to explode some of the stigma that stops people from asking questions and talking openly about all things vagina, the same stigma that made me think my vagina was broken for fourteen years. It should not be controversial showing a vulva or saying the word 'vagina', but every day people are shamed and censored for doing just this. Sadly, the only thing more shameful than having a vagina, it seems, is having one that doesn't do exactly what it says on the tin.

I often find penetrative sex painful.

I've been pussy (wheyo!) footing around writing that sentence for a little while, but there it is.

The act that is meant to be one of the most pleasurable, intense, passionate birthrights of being human for me can feel quite the opposite. It can sting. It can feel awkward, sometimes it just won't be possible at all. Vagina says no, you shall not pass! This can make me feel broken: as a lover, as a woman, as a human being. Alongside that . . .

I find it difficult to orgasm.

I want to be an overflowing bubbling brook of sexual vivacity, coming when the lightest breeze touches my skin. Nicki Minaj demands an orgasm every single time she has sex! I'm not asking for quite that much (although good on you, Nicki!), I just want sex to feel a bit nice some of the time. Disclaimer: I *can* orgasm. It *does* happen. For me, orgasm can take a level of concentration and time that drains the fun out of any sexual experience, leaves everyone's fingers bent in odd directions and the end results can be like a party popper that's been left in a garden shed for too

long. A few years ago though, I decided I wanted to fix this. My
mission to mend my broken vagina began.

Lots of people had opinions about my wanting to do this.

PEOPLE WITH OPINIONS: You're being a bit greedy Fran.

They were worried that like a sexy Icarus I might melt
my vulva right off through too much self-exploration.

PEOPLE WITH OPINIONS: Can't you just be pleased with
what your body *can* do? Rather than focusing on what it *can't*!
So negative!

I found myself apologising and feeling guilty for not feeling satisfied.

PEOPLE WITH OPINIONS: Where will it end Fran? Where
will it end?

It was nice they were concerned about me, but I wasn't sure
what they were afraid of. Surely the best-case scenario was that it
would end with more pleasure, more sexual satisfaction and more
confidence knowing that I had the right to *more*. Worst case
scenario was RSI and a slightly better understanding of my body.
Some research shows that in the workplace women are four times
less likely to ask for a raise in salary and when they do ask for one
it is for 30% less than men ask for.[1] I wondered if the same was
true of sex. Had I been conditioned to accept my lot, be grateful,
amiable, inoffensive, passive and never ask for more?
We as a species have mastered flight, transplanted the human

face and brought woolly mammoth cells back to life. How can we have a theory of quantum mechanics but still only 65% of heterosexual women orgasm most of the time during sex, compared to 95% of men?[2] Why is Viagra now available over the counter in UK pharmacies, whereas the equivalent for people with vaginas is either popping a crystal or a $1,500 injection into your genitals? Why, when we can make bionic eyes, is questioning a doctor about sex still often resulting in flustered paper shuffling? Why have there only been 5,000 publications on female sexual difficulties, compared to 14,000 on male sexual disorders?[3] Why were 99.99% of my sexual experiences framed by my partners' erection to ejaculation bookend? I felt I was owed a lot of answers (and a lot of orgasms).

My symptoms come under the umbrella diagnosis of FSD, Female Sexual Dysfunction, the sexiest of all the dysfunctions. This disorder can include problems with desire, orgasm and pain during sex, I have experienced all three of these at some point. According to the Sexual Advice Association, it is estimated around a third of young and middle-aged women suffer from a form of sexual dysfunction, along with around half of older women.[4] That is SO MANY people, but frighteningly probably only the tip of the iceberg, given it's not always a subject people openly discuss or feel comfortable seeking help for. I myself discovered the term while Googling my symptoms, trying to work out what exactly was wrong with me – and there it was (underneath many pop-up adverts for 'horny women in my area') Female Sexual Dysfunction.

Labels can be useful, it means the thing you are experiencing exists, you aren't going mad and it isn't all in your head. The word 'dysfunction' didn't sit well with me. It made me feel like a faulty vending machine, stuck half-way through releasing a KitKat. It made me want to take my vagina back to the shop for a refund immediately. I couldn't see myself reclaiming the condition, doing park runs wearing FSD wristbands or putting it on my dating profile, #sexuallydysfunctional #dysfunctionalfemale. If I was dysfunctional, surely I could be made functional? A technician could be called, I could be rebooted, turned off and back on again.

This book is for anyone who has ever put someone else's needs in front of their own, told a lie to save another's feelings or felt like they were doing something very basic very wrong. It's for anyone who has ever faked an orgasm, experienced pain or discomfort during sex (75% of women) or had their body in the room but their mind distracted thinking about the human rights of robots or the fact that there is plastic at the bottom of the seven-mile-deep Mariana Trench.[5] It is particularly for anyone who has been made to feel they are not sexually 'normal'.

I promise you are not on your own.

I have only ever had one vagina. I am a cisgender female and have only had sex with people who identify as male. I only know what it's like to have my vagina. I have no idea what it's like to have genitals that don't feel like they belong to my body. I have never given birth. I menstruate (irregularly, when my uterus feels like doing it – usually just as I hand over the cash to buy a pregnancy test). My experience is limited. No two humans are the same; no two sexual experiences are the same; no two vaginas are the same; some women don't have vaginas; some men do. I don't have a qualification in sex and I have absolutely no medical training (my last first aid certificate expired in 2004). I haven't even slept with *all* of the people to be able to give you a completely fair and thorough evaluation of *all* of the sex. I wish I could say go sleep with *so and so* from

Chichester and they'll sort it out, but I can't. I've just had some of the sex with some of the people and a bit with myself. To make sure my mission to fix my broken vagina was comprehensive and inclusive, I spoke to experts in sexual health, medicine and pleasure and asked strangers of all ages and backgrounds to generously share their own stories. Their stories appear as follows, alongside their age, if they wanted to share this.

Can you tell me something brilliant about your genitals?

My flaps are super stretchy. Me and a friend came home drunk once and showed each other how far they come out. 23

I can fanny fart on command, it's my party trick. 37

When I was 13, I found my clitoris and burnt it out during GCSE revision :-) 27

I put a tampon up my butt the first time I tried to use it. Then I had to use a pocket mirror for ages to find out where 'the right hole is'. 30

Can you tell me something brilliant about your genitals? was also the question that most people chose to skip or said things like . . .

No. And that's a bit sad. 41

Sadly, I can't think of anything. 23

I feel sad that I don't have anything to say here. 33

Statements such as '*I actually like the look of my genitals. 28*', should not have felt as radical, profound and rare as they did.

Collecting this information felt oddly rebellious. When I first attempted to get my questionnaire beyond my immediate generally sex-positive bubble, I found myself removed and banned from forums . . .

THREAD DELETED: Hard to explain why but when someone starts a thread containing the word 'Vagina' we become instantly suspicious.

Given unsolicited advice . . .

OMG you are a very confused woman! Sex is actually much simpler . . . you are just overthinking it. Just lie on your back and relax and enjoy

And made some *friends* along the way . . .

I bet you've got a fanny like a clown's pocket

Isn't the internet lovely?

A few wondered why I was asking to speak to 'people with vaginas', rather than using the term 'women'. Having a vagina doesn't make you a woman and being a woman doesn't mean you have a vagina. In my mind if you considered yourself to have a vagina, whatever meaning that had for you, I wanted to hear from and amplify your experience. As a straight, white cisgender woman I knew I had experienced enough difficulty being heard and listened to about my vagina; further silencing of voices certainly was and still is not what is needed. Language *is* important. Choice of words is powerful. I will be using the words 'female' and 'woman' when it pertains to my experience (because this is how I identify) and in quoting research studies and medical instances, where gender is currently documented as largely binary.

At times I felt like giving up on sex, because it often seemed like it wasn't for me. What kept me going was talking to other people about it, learning how intimacy fitted into their lives and how sex really isn't just the in-out in-out activity we learn about (if we are lucky) in Biology class. So, as well as the survey findings, throughout this book are interviews with people with different relationships to sex, talking candidly about their own experiences. I hope you will enjoy how there really is no such thing as 'normal'.

Some of my experiences described in this book are upsetting and others reading them might find them so. At the time I thought those experiences were 'just what modern dating is like'; I know now this isn't the case. At the back of this book is a list of organisations that offer support and information for anyone who finds themselves in a relationship they are struggling to get out of, and also for anyone who wants to ask for help with a sexual issue.

In writing this book I spent long days learning about sex, overthinking sex, reading sex facts, sex techniques, pouring over my own sexual history and solidifying and challenging my sexual beliefs and boundaries and then I'd slip into bed and try to uphold everything I'd learnt. Reader, I imagine having sex with me at that time was a bit like shagging a biology textbook (and a psychology textbook and sociology and probably a few other –ologies, no one needs to be told sex facts mid-coitus).

Knowledge is power but being too academic and serious about sex can disconnect you from your body all over again. So, breathe in, be ridiculous, be messy, be curious.

I wish I could guarantee incredible sex and an orgasm just from reading this book, imagine that! Bestseller list here I come (no pun intended . . . ok, maybe a small pun intended). Orgasms are not our goal here. I hope it creates some comfort in a world where talking about vaginas and their pleasure and pain is difficult, and often treated as novelty, invisible or frivolous. Feeling that a part of you is broken can be an incredibly lonely experience, so I hope more than anything this book can be a big reminder that no matter what your relationship with vaginas, you are absolutely not on your own.

I

Faking Orgasms & 'Is It My Penis?' Man

Yes! Yes! Yes!

This story began astride an ex-boyfriend.

Oh my. Right there. That's it.

I was twenty-nine years old and giving an Oscar award winning performance. Running my hands through my tangled hair, writhing passionately, I tossed my head frantically like an orca whale breaching the surface. Splash!

Yeehaaa. Ring-a-ding-ding. Wham Bam Thank You—

Through hair flicks and exuberant groans, I looked down proudly. He was absolutely loving this show. I was so good at being good at sex, an intercourse entertainer, a true coitus artiste.

I'm so close. I'll be coming round the mountain when I come. In 100 yards (according to satnav) I will have reached my destination.

I could almost imagine the trailer: 'Sex superstar Bushe gives a captivating and glamorously spellbinding performance in the sensual extravaganza of the year! Coming soon! Rated 18'

I had carefully curated this experience for him, so he could have no doubt at all that he was indeed an exceptional lover, THE BEST AT SEX, deserving of a gold medal and a place on the fourth plinth in Trafalgar Square.

He couldn't know what was really going on behind the scenes: pain, discomfort, a growing feeling of failure, all wrapped up in a real desire to give him the sexual experience he deserved. I had to hide the fact that his girlfriend of six months' vagina was broken. I knew that the louder and more exuberant I was, the more aroused he would become, the quicker he would orgasm and the sooner we could get to the bit I loved – the post-coital spooning and debrief of how nice the sex was (with me ignoring the ache between my legs). Besides, I was getting a lot of enjoyment from giving him a lovely time and maybe, just maybe that was enough.

RIGHT THERE! RIGHT THERE! RIGHT THERE!

Except for as I bobbed around on top of him, giving the full porn star experience, it just wasn't enough. It felt empty and, in the time it took me to notice I *really* was not enjoying it, I realised I'd been silent too long. It had been ages since I've made a sexy moan, so I refocused my performance, recommitted, with my brain giving directorial notes.

MY MOUTH: *OOOOOH!*
MY BRAIN: Mm too loud, he'll know you're compensating for being quiet so long.
MY MOUTH: *Oh!*

MY BRAIN: Too surprised, gentler, use your
diaphragm, work from your core.

MY MOUTH: *Erghhahaaahhaaaahh!*

MY BRAIN: Beautiful work Fran, very organic, a real
virtuoso performance.

MY MOUTH: *Wowee!*

MY BRAIN: He looks like he is having such a lovely
time.

MY MOUTH: *COR BLIMEY GUVNOR!*

MY BRAIN: I wish I was having a lovely time.

MY MOUTH: *Cabin crew prepare doors for landing!*

MY BRAIN: What's wrong with me? What's wrong
with my body? What's wrong with my vagina?

MY MOUTH: *YOU'RE THE BEST AT SEX!*
YOU'RE THE BEST AT SEX!

It is not a good feeling to resent the person whose penis is
inside you. It is not a good feeling to begrudge the person you
love their good time, but his and my experiences of that same
moment of sex could not have been further apart.

I tried to think about the things I *do* enjoy about sex by list-
ing them: the close intimacy, his breath on my skin, the smell,
accidentally seeing moving bodies reflected in a nearby mirror,
looking forward to wrapping myself in a blanket afterwards and
waddling to the bathroom trying not to splash on the carpet/
lino (depending if we are at his house or mine). If sex could be
more waddling, then wonderful. But that isn't what sex is. Sex
is connecting by the hips. Sex is supposed to be penetration
plus two orgasms (his and mine). No exceptions.

'Come for me' he said, an authoritative orgasm magician.
'Come for me' like it was just a switch you flick on. It would

have been rude not to though, especially when he had asked so nice and politely.

As he sped up, I spotted the visual clues that he was approaching orgasm. He zoned out and it felt like he was suddenly ready for his close-up and had decided he could play both lead characters, leaving me to be an extra in my own sex life.

I prepared my well-observed coming face: realistic and raw and very *very* unattractive (because it had to seem really *real*). Then maybe for the hundredth time in slow motion we *somehow* coincidentally managed to climax at *exactly* the same time. Moaning loudly together in a crescendo of love and forgery I told him, 'That was amazing!' and lay back on the sheets pretending to cinematically pant.

Beneath the recently buffeted bedsprings were boxes I'd picked up from my parents' house, filled with scraps of teenage nostalgia. One box contained endless blurry photographs of me in a parka with a swooping fringe, festival wrist bands I'd sworn I'd never cut off, cinema ticket stubs for *Love Actually*, *The Matrix Reloaded* and *How to Lose a Guy in 10 Days* – and box after box of diaries. I have nearly always kept diaries, voraciously as a teenager and sporadically ever since. Before rolling into bed that evening for this great sex performance, I'd flicked through the diaries of 16-year-old me in 2003 and read lines I'd written like . . .

My crush told me today that he is an Aquarius which makes him a whole 14 months older than me. That's surely too old don't you think? It's SUCH a big age gap . . .

And

Jay has decided to not talk to me today because of what we wrote on MSN last night. She has informed me she will resume speaking to me tomorrow at 9am . . .

And

I am thinking of getting a tattoo of a dolphin and some words in French in italics underneath . . . maybe J'adore?

Among all the teenage anxiety, friendship dramas and attempts at tiny rebellions I read . . .

I'm sure sex will get better. Things are always hard at first but get easier with time. Right? I bet it won't be long before I'm having AMAZING sex, every single time. Probably.
Tried crimping my hair today, but got bored halfway through, it is not as easy as Kim makes it look. I have a LOT of hair.

I'd sat and reread that diary entry over and over. Things hadn't gotten better, for sex (or my hair). Over a decade-and-a-half after writing that, lying there basking in *his* post-coital glow I couldn't shake an empty feeling. Sex hadn't gotten easier. I had failed 16-year-old Fran.

'How was that for you?' he asked smoothly. I opened my mouth to answer, but left too long a pause. Something in the elastic of myself snapped and I started to cry. I'd done this performance too many times and I'd forgotten my lines.

'Was is *that* good?' he asked hopefully. In *his* defence he had just witnessed an outstanding performance of sexual enjoyment (complete with standing ovations and multiple requests for a sequel). In *my* defence, they were really heaving, pillow-soaking tears, clearly not happy tears. I really did have a good feeling about this man beside me and maybe, just maybe, I thought he would be different. You see, by this point I'd been faking enjoyment of sex on and off for around fourteen years: it had become the norm. I had bad experiences of telling the truth.

'I really enjoy having sex with you,' I said delicately, 'But I find it really hard to orgasm and sex can be painful. I feel very broken *a lot* of the time. I always have I think.' Laying this truth out on the cotton sheets between us, I was completely honest about sex for the first time in six months. He stared at the ceiling contemplatively, breathing calm and easy. 'Maybe *he* will be different,' I hoped, 'Maybe this time will be different.'

After a few moments he turned his head to me, looked deep into my eyes and asked . . .

'Is it my penis?'

(It was not his penis).

'I thought I had a good penis. I've been told I have a really good penis.'

'It's really not your penis, you have a lovely penis . . . Go Penis!'

'I've always been considered *very* good at sex,' he added.

Cool.

'In fact, and I'm not one to brag, I have given *several* partners, multiple partners, their first ever orgasm. People who have NEVER come before. Never.'

Great. That's nice. I mean it did sound a little like bragging.

'I've never had any complaints, so, I just don't know what's *suddenly* wrong with *my* penis. What's wrong with *my* penis?'

He didn't stop saying the word penis at regular intervals for a long time.

'Penis . . . penis . . . penis . . . *penis* . . . *PENIS?!* . . . penis'.

I wanted to take back what I had just said, to cover this man in sexual medals and sky-write that he was one noteworthy lover in one-hundred-foot letters across the horizon. I patted his back, soothing his emotions.

'It's me that's broken,' I said, '*You* are great . . . *you* are perfect . . . your penis [kisses fingers extravagantly like a Michelin Star chef] so nice! What a lovely penis! Just the best of all peni.' He didn't hear me though and before I knew it, I'd decided it was too much honesty and maybe if I worked fast I could undo the damage.

'I'm just a bit of a mess today, hormones probably, period is very due, and my head just wasn't *in* the sex. Sorry, the sex *is* always really great, you are *really* great at sex, the best.'

I often dismiss and blame moments of sadness or anger on hormones. Sometimes it definitely is my hormones, oh boy is it my hormones, but not always. Sometimes the anger or sadness is what I am feeling, but don't feel allowed to say or express it, so my hormones take the blame. An hour later, he was still sitting looking damningly at his crotch like it had let the side down, penis and ego both flaccid. I decided to cheer him up. What really cheers him up? *Sex* really cheers him up.

'I'm sorry, I wasn't thinking about what I was saying, I love having sex with you, in fact-' I leant in, kissed him and . . . off we went. This time I was his full-time cheerleader, each moan erasing his memory: '*Oh, oh, oh,* forget what I just said, *yes, yes, yes,* you are such a talented lover, *that's the ticket.*'

As he finished, he looked at me eagerly.

'Did it work *that* time?'

I smiled.

'You are the best at sex.'

19

He fell asleep and I pressed my thighs together, trying to numb the pain, feeling like an idiot.

Throughout my twenties I had tried to be honest with partners, but they had seen my 'difficulty' to enjoy sex as a failing on their part (or parts). When I was honest with them, the truth then lay in bed with us like a strange ménage à trois, impossible for us to ignore or get past. I had come to the point of believing that it wasn't possible to be in a happy relationship with a broken vagina, so the choice was either lie about enjoying sex or be alone.

Neither 'Is It My Penis?' Man nor I behaved perfectly in this. I know now that for him realising that I'd been lying about my experience of sex for months will have felt like a betrayal, adding doubt to a situation where you are meant to be at your most connected and vulnerable with someone. So, I think there's space here for an apology . . .

Dear ex-lovers,

I'm sorry I wasn't completely honest with you about sex.

Often when I told the truth you closed down and thought it was a personal critique of 'your moves'. I should have been honest, but pride, fear of rejection, and sometimes even love was wrapped up in there too, so I stopped telling you it hurt, because it hurt *you* too much. In the future, if someone should happen to feel courageous enough to share with you, know that it isn't an attack or a complaint. So please be kind.

Lots of love and thanks for all the spooning,

Fran x

I lay in bed next to a sleeping 'Is it My Penis?' Man, feeling like a failure. Failing him by not responding to his touch *properly*. Failing feminism and womankind, because this is the twenty-first century and I should have been an advocate for my own pleasure and not just be a penis pleaser. And failing myself, why was my body so bad at being a body? My mind kept me awake with an incessant and highly critical inner monologue.

> MY BRAIN: This is your fault Fran, you should tell him what is and isn't working, he isn't a mind reader for heaven's sake! How is he meant to drive the car without a road map?
> ME: I don't even know how to drive the car, I'm not even sure where it's parked, I think I've lost the car keys!
> MY BRAIN: You are behaving like a wank sock Fran!

I didn't enjoy feeling like a wank sock.

Advice columns say, 'Just tell them what you need!', like this is the simplest of sex moves, but when I was with someone I cared about deeply, or even a brand-new partner who I wanted to like me, it wasn't always that easy. It wasn't even straightforward knowing what I needed or wanted in the first place. At other times I had said what I needed loud and clear, but being heard and listened to was something different altogether.

Have you ever exaggerated enjoyment of sex?

I would (almost) always fake enjoyment. I thought that if I didn't enjoy sex that would mean I was boring, and then men wouldn't like me. Even though I know it's a stupid thing to do and that it doesn't help anyone, I sometimes still fake enjoyment, just to keep my partner happy. 32, f

Yes. To try and give my partner encouragement and confidence. During the 25 years I was with my husband, I frequently put up with things that weren't quite right and made me cringe. I would try and sound calm and positive while inside I was screaming with frustration. 50, f

Yes – he told me he was good at sex, so I just assumed that I was in the wrong! 27, f

Yes. I think it was a pressure of knowing how porn sounds and worrying I was broken that I wasn't making the right sounds. Always about them and ensuring their ego knew I had a *really* great time after, thanks. 28, f

Sometimes a bit so I looked like a free and sexually advanced liberated fully self actualised kind of woman who orgasms all the time and easily so they would say 'wow she is just so free and comfortable with herself!' 36, f

There was so much care, love and self-sacrifice in many of the survey answers I read. People putting their own experience and pleasure as secondary to their partner, not wanting to upset people they cared about, hiding pain because they felt it was their fault. So many people felt like their role in sex was to be enjoyed and provide enjoyment . . . rather than to enjoy the experience themselves.

Have you ever faked an orgasm and why?

Yes. Wanting sex to be over. Politely. 41, f

Yes. Because sometimes sex hurts, or it isn't fun, or what's fun for your partner isn't fun for you. There's a pressure to really enjoy penetrative sex, it's not socially acceptable to admit sex is sometimes naff. 29, f

While my partner was certainly putting a lot of effort into making sure I finished, after a certain point it becomes painful and I wanted him to stop without hurting his feelings. 25, f

Yes. To keep my marriage alive. 50, f

Among the answers that describe exaggerating pleasure as just the expected thing and looking after a partner's experience, there were also suggestions that sounding like you were having a really fabulous time, can help make you feel more aroused and may make it more likely that you will orgasm.

Fake it till you make it sometimes works for me, faking can increase my arousal and then lead to a real orgasm. 40, f

Oh yeah, loads of times, but performing over the top enjoyment or arousal is also hot in my opinion. For the enjoyment and fun for everyone involved honestly. 30, gender-fluid

The 'fake it till you make it' method (if I act or sound turned on, it helps them feel turned on, which helps ME feel turned on. If that makes sense lol). 22, f

It isn't in itself a bad thing to exaggerate here and there, especially if it is feeding into your own sexual confidence and enhancing your own arousal. But when it becomes a consistent strategy, a buffer, a bartering tool or a gift then we should perhaps ask ourselves, who is our orgasm for and wouldn't it just be nicer if we had a real one? Why are we so scared of the silence that would be there if we didn't exaggerate and pretend (easy for me to say, I wouldn't cope well with the silence at all, I'd probably start humming or debating or reciting a poem to fill the void). If the 'ooohs' and 'aaahs' and 'yes, right there's' are filling the space of an honest conversation about our enjoyment of sex then perhaps we need a rethink.

Having an orgasm definitely shouldn't be the marker of a successful sexual experience. The goal orientated pressure of sex, the striving to finish, to cross the line, to see the fire-works display at the end can make being in the moment and enjoying sex harder. I have also been told many, many times that the best way to have an orgasm is to try and not have one. There are people who practise the art of Karezza or Coitus Reservatus, where couples consciously take orgasm off of the table, focusing instead on touch, slow sex and connection. However, if you do want to have one, then wonderful.

I thought back over what teenage Fran had written in her diary.

I'm sure sex will get better, these things do, right? They are always hard at first but get easier with time. Right?

I felt I owed her something better. She had been so hopeful and so sure that she was just at the start of things.

Lying next to a sleeping 'Is it My Penis?' Man, I picked up a half full diary from under the bed, found a new blank page, grabbed a pen and wrote:

New Rules for Sex

NO MAKING SEX NOISES – No emitting sounds like the ones you hear in porn, or in films or from late night foxes shagging in gardens. Any noise I make must arise from actual pleasure I feel OR be turning me on sufficiently that it's enhancing the experience FOR ME.

NO PULLING SEX FACES – Unless they pull themselves. No gurning, no lip biting, no contorting my mouth into expressions of pure feigned ecstasy.

NO FAKING ORGASM – No pretending that I've finished or even that I'm close. From now on only total honesty. If I'm asked, 'Are you close?' I will say . . . 'No. Not at all. Not even in the right postcode'.

LEARN WHAT I LIKE – Because at this point besides making a partner happy, I didn't have a clue.

* * *

Turn-Ons & Turn-Offs

While writing this book, I really threw myself into trying to discover what I enjoy sexually. I dived in headfirst, lube in hand, with mood music playing into the sexual unknown. Sometimes I pushed myself vastly outside of my comfort zone, sometimes it was much quieter simpler tasks, involving just spending time with my body (which in truth I found a whole lot harder). I learnt a lot of little things along the way that I'd like to share with you at the end of each chapter. They won't all be for everyone (drawing your own vulva probably *isn't* for everyone), but hopefully there might be something useful, like a pick-and-mix of sexual exploration.

The first tip I'd like to share is working out what turns you on and off. Sex had always been for the other person and so I had to tune into what actually made *me* feel good and I didn't know where to start. *Come as You Are* by Emily Nagoski was the first book that made me feel like maybe I wasn't sexually broken. In it she describes how important context is to a sexual experience. Context can be anything from emotional, environmental or romantic, to whether or not you are wearing socks. Fun fact: wearing socks allegedly does make it more likely that people with vaginas will orgasm, so I'll be keeping my socks on forevermore . . . the warmer and woollier the better.[6]

Nagoski describes the dual control model of sexual response, developed by Erick Janssen and John Bancroft in the late 1990s: our brains are always scanning our surroundings for reasons to be turned on (accelerators) and reasons that being aroused might not be for the best at that exact moment (brakes). Some people have more sensitive accelerators and some have more sensitive brakes. For some people sex in public might be the ultimate thrill, while for others it might be a massive no thanks; we are all different. She encourages people to think about enjoyable sexual experiences they've had and notice (in detail) what the context was, in a bid to try and define what helps us become aroused. To do this I started keeping a record of things that made me feel sexual and more likely to have a good experience.

These were some of the things I noticed about myself.

Accelerators

- Having enough time. Not snatched moments between answering emails and having to leave to catch the bus.
- Scents. I enjoy smells, every so often I'll stop still on the street because I'll walk past someone who smells like my first ever boyfriend's deodorant. Seducing my nostrils is important. Candles are also great.
- To feel completely safe – encompassing and ranging from the door being properly closed (yes, I will get out of bed several times to check it is secure) to a certainty that the relationship is doing ok.

Brakes

- A stressful day. Ruminating on thoughts is an enormous sensuality killer for me, I just can't keep my mind in the room if I am fretting.
- Not feeling clean.
- Having other people in the house, I worry any noise will disturb them

I think in the past I've often felt the things I need to get me in the mood are unsexy, overly romantic or boring. I wanted to be able to be the person who can pull a partner into a stationery cupboard for a quickie . . . but realistically I would need hours of relaxing against the photocopier and a candle perching on the fax machine first. Seeing the things I need written down on paper made me realise this is just where I am at, at the minute. It doesn't mean I will insist a candle is lit every time I have sex, that might become oddly Pavlovian and could get awkward on people's birthdays. But if I know there isn't going to be time for me to be properly relaxed, I'll just say 'Let's do this later'. If I was worrying about something, I'd ask to talk the worry through to clear my mind.

Easy right?

HONEST CONVERSATIONS ABOUT SEX
Sex is like dancing

A: woman, lesbian, she, 57
B: woman, lesbian, she, 57

A: We met dancing!

B: I had decided to go out and do something fun, so I went women-only ballroom dancing.

A: I am not a ballroom dancer. I had been married to a man, I came out later in life and was in the process of divorcing. I'd been in the closet for a long time, but it'd been bubbling under the surface. The sexual side was not a happy place for me in my marriage, and as time went on I realised I shouldn't be with a man. I had issues of painful sex, not at the beginning of the relationship but the more I realised it wasn't right for me, definitely.

B: Just to give a contrast, I came out in my 20s, I had lots of boyfriends before and loved sex with them. In my second year of uni, me and my boyfriend went to watch a porno . . . *Emmanuelle 2* and there's this bit of girl-on-girl action. Emmanuelle was in the forest in Thailand, she met this blonde strapping archeologist and they got it on and I thought 'Oh . . . my . . . god' . . . Let's just say that night I was really, really turned on.

A: I've never really enjoyed sex with men but I just hadn't worked out why. I always felt like it was me, something wrong with me. I couldn't orgasm with a man. In my marriage the only way I could orgasm was to masturbate myself. Sex was penetrative, that's all I knew about.

B: You don't have any hang-ups about masturbation and that gave me permission to not feel sad about it. I used to feel 'Oh I shouldn't be doing this' or 'I'm only doing this because I don't have anyone' but I don't feel that with you.

A: Masturbation has kept me going over the years. I don't think it's anything naughty, it's something that's really important, a very positive thing.

B: In terms of masturbation while making love I wasn't sure at first but then we talked about it and the way we get to orgasm is different. It's the general sort of friction for me whereas you have to be very focused and in a particular rhythm. At the beginning learning to touch you, I was feeling like 'I don't know how to play this song' or 'this is a blues song but I'm playing it as a jazz song'. Sometimes it's much easier for you to play your own song.

A: We've taken what I'd have thought of as sex and blown that up.

B: I'm excited that we are in our 50s and rediscovering a beautiful, intense sexual relationship. Sex is like dancing; it's about having *that* connection and playing with each other and being with each other in the moment. If we danced mechanically, 'This goes here and this will lead to this', there would be no chemistry.

A: I don't remember sex being painful in my 20s, I wasn't really into it and . . . you don't mind me talking about this do you? I think in my heart of hearts it was a psychology thing. People ask me how I didn't know I was a lesbian growing up and I just didn't, I didn't have exposure to it.

B: Since menopause it hurts and no matter if I'm turned on and—

A: Very lubricated—

B: Only once were you able to go in. It's very frustrating, because I feel like I want it, but when you've tried it, it doesn't work . . . but being gay, penetrative sex has never been a huge thing, so I've always had pleasure from clitoral stimulation, it just occurs to me it must be much harder in a straight relationship because sex can equal penetration.

A: I'm proud that we talk about our sex life in the same way we talk about what we are going to have for supper.

B: We are older ladies but having more sex than anyone I can think of.

2

Dirty Thirties & The Guide to Sex

<u>New Rules for Sex</u>
NO MAKING SEX NOISES
NO PULLING SEX FACES
NO FAKING ORGASM
LEARN WHAT YOU LIKE

I was cheating a bit when I made myself those rules lying next to a sleeping 'Is It My Penis?' Man. I knew I wouldn't really need to do or change much for this sexual awakening to happen. That was because something momentous was approaching, something that would effortlessly revolutionise my relationship with my body and set fire to my sex life. I was days away from (drumroll, please) . . . turning thirty. Cue fireworks; cue laser show; cue full orchestra playing 'Happy Birthday to Fran'.

I was knocking on the door of the decade affectionately named the 'dirty thirties'. The prophesied sexual awakening, my foretold (by *Sex and the City* and glossy magazines) sexual peak was almost upon me. This societal understanding was largely born from the 1950s' Kinsey Reports by zoologist Alfred Kinsey, which found that women had more orgasms in their thirties than at any other point in their lifetimes.[7] There is much of this study that has been deemed controversial (Kinsey interviewed and failed to report sex criminals) and a lot has changed since the 1950s (it was published before the introduction of the contraceptive pill, which fundamentally changed sexual habits), but the idea that the thirties are a fabulous decade for vaginas has clung on. In all reality, it is probable that sex is better in our thirties and beyond because we know our bodies better, feel more comfortable in them and are more likely to be in relationships, where statistically better sex is reported . . . either way I felt sure I was about to blossom.

When I told a scientist friend about the threshold I was about to cross he said:

SCIENCE FRIEND: Women are hornier in their thirties because their biological clock is ticking. It's nature's way of telling you to get on with it and procreate. Tick-tock.

I didn't like the idea that my promised sexual dawn would be the result of my body panicking about making mini-Frans. I'm also not a massive fan of anyone saying the phrase 'tick-tock' to me. All I knew was something would click into place inside of me and I'd be suddenly continuously aroused – titillated while grouting, horny while receiving a cold call for life insurance, orgasming eating Wotsits on the 147 bus. All I had to do was hold on, sail into my thirties, with 'Is it My Penis?' Man by my side. As I lay next to him, I knew excitedly I was about to begin my sexual odyssey, no more faking, only honesty. I was going to be orgasming my socks off (and back on again, because as we know, socks = more orgasms) very shortly.

'I think we should break-up,' Is it My Penis? Man said the next morning, as he plunged his coffee vigorously.

'Oh.'

So that was that.

My break-up at 29 isn't what this book is about. Not to minimise it at all (especially for anyone currently going through the bone-crushing pain of a break-up), I can assure you there was lots of crying, attempts at reconciliation (he'd change his mind back pretty much after he had orgasmed every time), loads of my being aloof in order to try and win him back with varying levels of success, weeks of crying everywhere I went (including several very important meetings and lots of long train rides), days of posting pictures on social media of me having an endlessly incredible (but very sad inside) time and writing terrible emotional poetry about my heart (luckily lots of things rhyme with pain). The most important thing about this is that once the fog of the break-up had thinned, I realised this was the perfect time for me to fix my broken vagina. I mean sure, I was days away from my thirtieth birthday, suddenly dumped and about to approach my sexual peak with no one to climb it with. Of course, all my peak-climbing goods and sexy Kendal mint cake were at risk of going soggy in my backpack, but without having another person's feelings to protect, I might actually – for perhaps the first time ever – be able to prioritise myself during sex. Imagine that.

Up until that point most of my sexual adventuring had happened within long-term relationships. I was suddenly not in one of those anymore. I had never had a one-night stand.

The truth is I found the idea of casual sex very difficult. Not morally. I loved the idea of making eye contact with someone across a room, walking over, telling them to get their hat, gloves and scarf for they have pulled and enjoying a one-night-only human-to-human connection (preferably in a barn or a deserted mill or on a pollen-free riverbank), but with my body comes a lot of sexual admin. If I wanted to have casual sex, I was going to have to have vulnerable conversations with complete strangers, when I already struggled to have those chats with people I really loved. Terrifying.

At what point on a date with someone new, do you say, 'Hey, I know we are probably going to go back to mine and bang it out/make sexy magic, but I want you to know . . . I might find this very painful and you will need to do a lot of foreplay, I mean A LOT. Your fingers are really going to ache and we need to do it in very specific positions for it to even be anywhere near comfortable for me, and the likelihood is I won't orgasm, so let's not go for too long else it will just start to chafe and hurt? In fact, should we just make some pancakes instead? Not a sexual euphemism, just actual crêpes.'

How do you say this without ruining the sexy mood you've spent the whole date cultivating? Mentioning this before you've started eating dinner feels presumptuous.

WAITER: And what would madame like to start?
ME: Oh, anything that will go with the very difficult
    sex we are going to have once we've eaten.
WAITER: The sea bass will go excellently with that.

Once you are actually in the bedroom seems likely to dampen or slow the moment.

THEM: Oh, I want you so much, sexy talk, sexy talk,
    sex sex sex!

ME: LET ME TELL YOU ABOUT MY BROKEN VAGINA . . .

Perhaps all of the sexual admin could be bundled into a text pre-date . . . but I appreciate it really is a lot to take on board before even meeting someone.

> THEM: Looking forwards 2 meeting u. 7 p.m.?
> ME: Perfect. Do you want to know about my [sad smiley face emoji] vag? [taco emoji].

The fear of having this conversation with a stranger not only meant I had never had a one-night stand, it also meant I'd stayed in bad relationships longer than I should, because I'd rather be in that sexual safety net of an unhappy relationship, than have to explain my vaginal know-how to someone new from scratch. The way I had sex in relationships was very far from perfect. I had tolerated unsatisfying sex in the past because I loved my partners deeply and had wanted a loving relationship above all other things (silly, silly love). I didn't know how to disconnect sex from love, because it was the love that kept me safe and buffered me when sex was painful and hard.

In an ideal world, I could whip out a fully animated PowerPoint presentation and project 'The Guide to Sex with Fran' on the bedroom ceiling, giving the required information without any of the awkward stuttering. Something so that when people ask 'What exactly is wrong with you Fran?' I could just click play and . . .

FRAN'S INSTRUCTIONAL GUIDE TO SEX

Hello you!

It is sexy time and you have been selected for some sex. Congratulations! The lights are low (potentially candles, but not so many that it seems like a fire hazard), the sex music playlist is playing and *we* are about to commence making love. Bow chicka wow wow.

Before we get 'down to it' there are a few things I'd like you to know.

Step one: MY BODY. Welcome to my body.

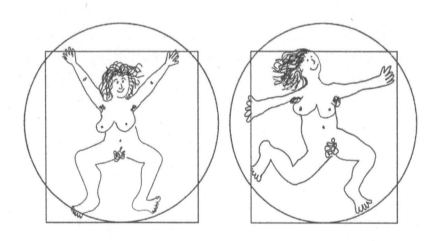

I will probably have been worrying about my body since before the date started. I mostly love my body, but when I think about it being naked in front of another person this may change. I will have tried to predict whether you like lots of pubic hair or no pubic hair (and potentially gone for some sort of panicky middle ground). I will be thinking about how to lie down so my breasts look pert-ish and will have chosen a posture that best hides my stretch marks. Women who feel negatively about their bodies often report lower levels of desire and arousal, decreased pleasure, orgasm and sexual satisfaction, which is unsurprising, because worrying about our bodies during sex is not a very sexy feeling.[8]

One bit of my body I particularly like is my sexy, sexy, sexy mind. Oh yeah baby! My mind is going to try and stay in the bedroom with you, but along with a whole host of body worries, it's going to be thinking about how we went to the petting zoo earlier for our date (very good choice of date you, well done) and you hand-fed that goat and now the hand that fed that goat is sliding down my body towards my vulva and all I'm thinking is:

GOAT HAND
GOAT HAND
GOAT HAND

But I'm also thinking about climate change.

And Michael Gove (Why?? Get out of my head Michael Gove! Now it's Michael Gove riding a goat! Begone Michael Gove and his sex goat!)

And wondering what does a spleen do anyway?

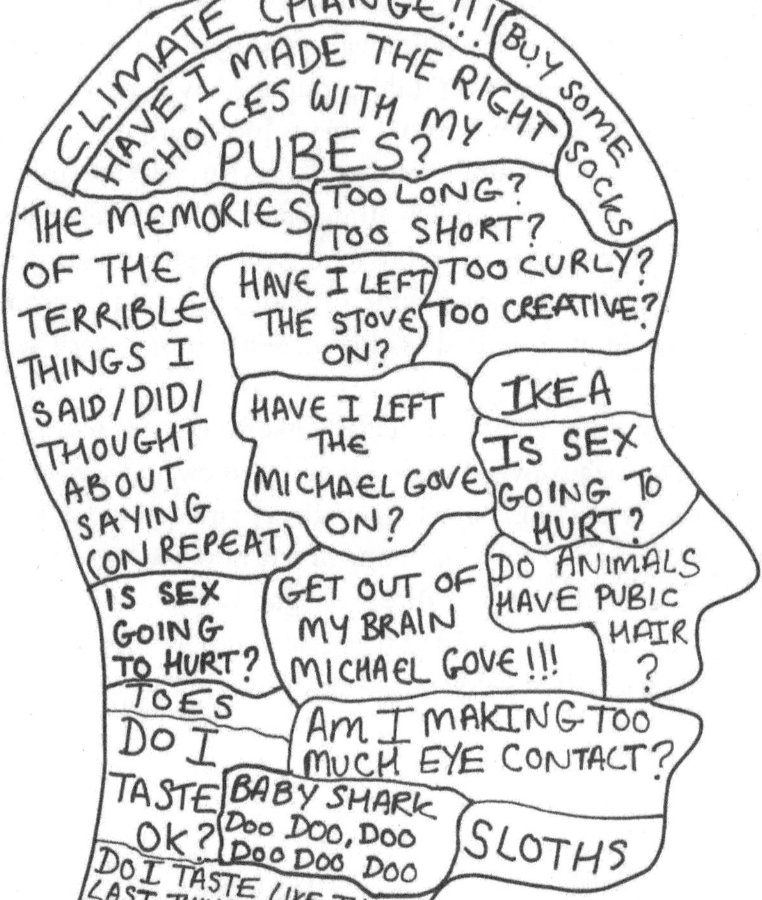
CLIMATE CHANGE!!!
BUY SOME SOCKS
HAVE I MADE THE RIGHT CHOICES WITH MY PUBES?
THE MEMORIES OF THE TERRIBLE THINGS I SAID/DID/THOUGHT ABOUT SAYING (ON REPEAT)
TOO LONG? TOO SHORT? TOO CURLY? TOO CREATIVE?
HAVE I LEFT THE STOVE ON?
HAVE I LEFT THE MICHAEL GOVE ON?
IKEA
IS SEX GOING TO HURT?
DO ANIMALS HAVE PUBIC HAIR?
IS SEX GOING TO HURT?
GET OUT OF MY BRAIN MICHAEL GOVE!!!
TOES
AM I MAKING TOO MUCH EYE CONTACT?
DO I TASTE OK?
BABY SHARK DOO DOO, DOO DOO DOO DOO
SLOTHS
DO I TASTE LIKE THE LAST THING I ATE? DO I TASTE LIKE MASHED POTATOES?
MAKE A SEX NOISE!!!!

I'm also mostly worrying about whether sex is going to hurt.

I've never known if sex hurts because I'm not turned on enough or I'm not turned on enough because I'm worrying sex is going to hurt! Over time that has become an unbreakable cycle, with worry about pain making me less turned on, which makes it more painful, which makes me less turned on, which makes it more painful . . . Oh baby, isn't this a sexy cycle?

The most sensitive part of my whole body is maybe my ears, but I am still working on a sexy way to say, 'Give me aural sex now, lick my lobes!'

Once we've done some awkward *elbow stuck in sleeve – should have taken shoes off before your trousers* – fumbling, it's time to welcome to the party: my vulva.

I don't want to leave my sex educator hat on too much in the bedroom, but I just think it's important that we always remember that the vulva is the external bit and the vagina is the internal bit.

Vulva = External. Vagina = Internal. Vulva = External. Vagina = Internal.

Pay attention lover, because there will be a quiz at the end.

WARNING: if you are getting up close and personal with my vulva just be aware there can be a slight debris zone, so anything that my vulva has been near that day can end up stuck in and around it. Fluff, string, door keys. If you lose your bookmark while reading this book, it may well be in my vulva.

If sex is going to hurt, it's going to hurt at [Point A] and that is because it is DRY DRY DRY.

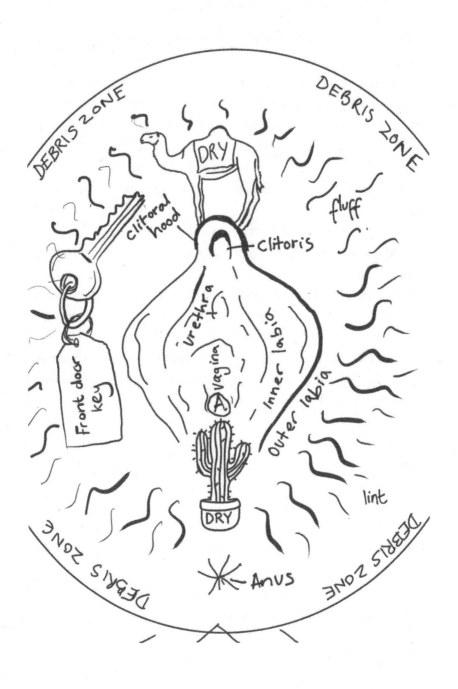

We can use lube, sure, but I'll be a bit embarrassed because you brought your penis AND an erection, the least I could do is be wet for you right? That's my job, I'm the host! I should provide chips, dip and endless natural lubrication. My vulva should be well presented, fragrant and exactly the correct room temperature (please feel free to leave your feedback in the visitors' book).

I'm sure this is really turning you on, right? This is getting you ready for sex!

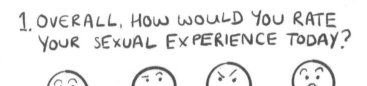

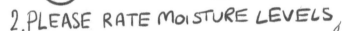

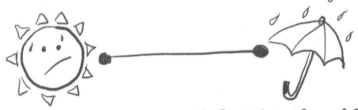

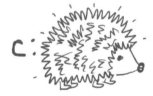

If you're going in, use a protractor for a clear 125-degree entry. The angle that makes it hurt less for me isn't a very friendly angle for a penis unfortunately. So, we'll do an awkward sort of barn dance manoeuvre, 'grab your penis by the hand and swing you round and do-si-do'! If we haven't entirely lost the moment and I actually manage to get you past the opening of my vagina (not guaranteed), I advise you to go steady at a speed of five TPM (Thrusts Per Minute) . . . (PS: in and out counts as TWO separate thrusts.)

If you get all the way inside (well done, team) watch out for my coil, this one is particularly pokey, numerous intrepid vagina explorers have complained they've been prodded by the end of it. For the most daring travelers, legend has foretold there is a G-spot (some say it exists, some say it doesn't; we can chat about it later); a U-spot (right by the urethra); a P-spot (on the posterior wall of the vagina); an A-spot (between the G-spot and the cervix) and a Wi-Fi hotspot (password required), but to be honest I'll probably ask you to stop before we get to any of those. Then it's time for a swift withdrawal, attention this vehicle is reversing, one hand firmly keeping condom in place as we both look intensely serious about not wanting to procreate in this exact moment.

I'll be available for a few minutes spooning and reflective feedback but then I'll need to go for a post-sex wee to avoid any UTI. (This is the best sex tip I was ever given. Perhaps urinary-tract infections could be added to sex education lessons at school? I've certainly had more dealings with UTIs than I have with the order of the planets . . . My Very Educated Mother Just Named the post-sex wee as the best way of avoiding UTIs. No matter how comfy you are, just wee!)

I'll probably be a bit sad after sex, because I'll have been very hopeful that *this* time might be better, this time might be THE ONE and I'll be angry and think that my vagina is the enemy. You might be a bit sad after sex, because you'll think it's your penis's fault. We'll sit there in a slump feeling angry at our genitals and I'm probably going to want sex a little less next time, and then a little less the time after that.

And maybe then a little less the next time after that.

And so on.

And so forth.

Um, so do you want to have sex with me and my broken vagina?

END OF FRAN'S INSTRUCTIONAL GUIDE TO SEX. Any questions?

Fourteen years earlier I had written in my teenage diary of my first love . . .

I just want to make him happy. I let him do things to me because it makes him happy. And it makes me happy to see him happy. How else will he be happy?

It was time for things to change.

* * *

Mindfulness

Mindfulness is the state of drawing attention and focus to thoughts, sensations and feelings in the present moment. I have always held the belief that I am bad at mindfulness. During a mindful practice something as simple as paying attention to my breath can spiral into continuous thoughts of 'I am terrible at this . . . I can't even breathe right . . . I am the worst of all breathers'. There's a mindfulness exercise where you pay close attention to a raisin rather than just shoving the raisin in your mouth: look at the raisin, smell the raisin, feel the raisins many ridges, savour the raisin . . . then eat the raisin. Every time I have attempted this, I have eaten the raisin way before I am asked to, only to look around the room and see everyone else still gazing lovingly at their raisin (and I don't even like raisins).

You've heard in this chapter how my mind can be flooded with other thoughts during sex. But what if a simple mind-fulness practice (one that didn't spiral into a tornado of me throwing a strop at my inability to be still and prematurely swallowing my raisin) was the key to helping my sex life.

In Lori A. Brotto's *Better Sex through Mindfulness: How Women Can Cultivate Desire*, it is reported that after an eight-session mindfulness programme sexual satisfaction for partici-pants increased by 60%.[9] That is a huge finding and my very stubborn brain would be an idiot not to give mindfulness a proper try. Research suggests that mindfulness can help with orgasms, sexual satisfaction, arousal and even experiencing pain during sex.[10] It also suggests that women can be fully aroused physically but sometimes just not be paying attention to it and therefore miss important sexual cues.[11] Even in highly arousing situations, sometimes our brains are so busy we miss the signs and signals in the world around us and our own bodies that we are turned on.

I'd been advised to practise being mindful outside of a sexual situation, so it could become a habit before I took it into a situation where there's a lot of other context (bodies, bushes and bits banging) to contend with. I found an audio version of a mindfulness practice, meant to be about slowing down, tuning in and being present. I was hoping it would help me bring my focus to my body and sensations (and make me a powerful sexual goddess for the coming day ... imagine a normal day but really sexy). For the first few minutes, I thought 'I am doing so well at this, I am absolutely brilliant at mindfulness, look at me go' and then that started to trickle into, 'Am I doing this right? I'm never going to get the hang of this. I am so peckish for a raisin right now.' This constant commentary during intimate moments can be called 'spectatoring' (a term coined by sex researchers Masters and Johnson), where you are essentially watching and critically assessing yourself.[12] It is not sexy. The recording told me that one of the most important things is to be non-judgemental and if I catch myself having a negative thought or feeling like my mind was wandering to just notice the thought and draw my mind back to my breath. I actually felt like I was starting to get the hang of it but midway through my mum popped her head round the door to tell me about a local riverside walk that's listed on the Merton Council website (an admittedly lovely stroll down the historic River Wandle!).

Once I was thinking about the riverside flora and fauna, it was hard to get my mind back on my body and breath. It served to remind me that getting the conditions right for intimacy is really hard. Living situations, work schedules and day-to-day life can make it sometimes feel impossible to take time for yourself. At the end of the exercise, I expected fast results but it served to remind me that this takes time, patience and practice.

HONEST CONVERSATIONS ABOUT SEX
Sex is pulling a face and quivering

Woman, bisexual, she/her, 23

Every time that you try to do research about sex and disability, there's so little about pleasure and fun and positivity, it is shocking how little there is out there.

We want to fuck.

For a long time, sex wasn't important to me at all. I'd gone to university and at this point my disability took over and became the entire focus of life, just coping with day-to-day living. I've now managed this year to prioritise my needs and my pleasure and sex has started to become important to me again.

Sex gives you a chance to be intimate and explore your body with different people. I found with my disability that means exploring other ways to enjoy my body and be pleasured. There is nothing better and more emotionally vulnerable than coming and pulling a face and quivering with somebody, to share the most inner part of yourself. I love it. I still manage to walk a bit of the time, but a lot of the time I'm a wheelchair user and a crutch user and a mobility aid user. The more we talk about disabled sex, the more representation and visibility there is, the more people can discover that they are not alone and that they can fuck all night long.

I love my body and everything that it does but it's taken time and therapy to get to this point, and sometimes I wish I could just be 'normal' but then I wouldn't be me, I wouldn't be this absolute unicorn of a human. I'm most proud of how I take control of my solo sex life, I'm really taking control of my pleasure and my ability to orgasm. I've never been one for wild partnered sex, I get off on kissing and touching and the feel of my body moving with somebody else, the build-up, all of that energy, is *bellissimo*! If you don't know about what you've got or where things are pleasurable in your vagina, where the ridges and dents are, what the cervix feels like, physically get in there with a mirror and have a good old root around.

Seventy per cent of able-bodied people said that they wouldn't have sex with a disabled person . . . I mean, what the fuck? It's really hard, especially in the disabled dating world, it can be a shit show for people being like 'By the way before we meet tomorrow, I'm a wheelchair user' and the other person saying like, 'Oh, this isn't going to work for me'.

Communication is the most important thing, it's so basic and everyone says it all the time but it's imperative to every part of sex. There is no formula, it can start differently every time, it can be anything, you've just got to be authentically yourself and live whatever experiences are right for you.

3

16-Year-Old Fran & Losing My Virginity

I didn't start life thinking my vagina was broken. As a child, I had an excellent anatomical understanding of my genitals.

It was obvious to me that I had TWO HOLES. Hole number one was called THE MINI (although it could equally be Minnie; I never saw it written down). This Mini/Minnie was for passing urine and also for babies. Despite its diminutive name, it was actually a large, bucket-shaped swirling void that babies would fall out of with ease. Plonk.

Hole number two was THE VAGINA (most commonly known as the anus). At primary school, a friend and I would don our imaginary white coats and take to our doctor's surgery in the bushes. Once fully hidden we would declare, 'There's something wrong with my mini and my vagina' . . . before prescribing the only medicine we knew of: a fresh leaf sandwiched between the buttocks. We then spent the rest of the school day with the rustle of foliage in our pants. Everything seemed present, correct and fun.

Let's just take a moment to lift our hats to five-year-old Fran for using an anatomical word, 'vagina', albeit entirely anatomically incorrectly. This was something I continued doing until my late twenties, except I called the whole area between my legs my vagina, or just nodded pointedly towards my crotch with a wink that I thought screamed 'VAGINA'. I strode around using the word as a vag of honour, proving my feminist credentials with each one of it's empowering sylla-bles: VA–GI–NA, VA–GI–NA. I was so proudly unafraid to say the word VAGINA, that I didn't even notice I was using the word completely incorrectly. I am not alone in this, as a study in 2016 showed that 70% of women could correctly identify the foreskin, penis and testes but 60% couldn't iden-tify the vulva and 45% the vagina.[13] Now in my thirties, after having had both body parts for all this time, I know that – let me hear you say it – the vagina is internal and the vulva is external.

Can you share your first memory of having a vulva or vagina? (Even if these weren't the words you were using for them at the time).

When I was four, I thought of my labia as tiny curtains to a theatre stage and made them 'open and close'. 22

Watching The X-Files *as a kid and getting turned on by the main guy and experiencing a 'feeling' down there.*

I think I was about three when I realised I had a 'front bottom' instead of a 'sausage bottom'. 30, f

I read a book at twelve about a girl masturbating, poked my finger in there and was like 'This doesn't live up to the hype'. 27, f

My vulva and vagina caused me relatively few worries until I hit my teenage years. Let's take ourselves back to 2003 and that teenage diary of mine. I'm sixteen years old, *Dawson's Creek* has just ended and The Darkness seem like a band that will go on and on forever. Teenage Fran believes in a thing called love and thinks that sex will be like the women in the Herbal Essences adverts, coming exuberantly under waterfalls, with Leonardo DiCaprio leaning on a moss-covered rock nearby and Sarah Michelle Geller dipping one *very* curious toe into my mountain stream.

PS: I haven't changed a word of this.

> *Dear diary,*
>
> *Me and Lee had some serious chats and decided that we were both ready to take our relationship to the next level. So, I went down on him. It is very rewarding to be able to do something like that for your loved one and for them to really enjoy it. Upon writing this in hindsight I'm unsure if I ought to have done it as now it feels like it is all I do and I am beginning to get a sore neck. The difference is he is for sure far more AHEM turned on by it and I can bring him to AHEM climax every single time. But I don't think I've ever been close. This of course isn't his fault as I'm unsure I will ever be 'turned on', I'm just as I told him not wired up right. But this is not important – physicality isn't important – I love his company and that is all that matters to me. Yesterday we went to the football and after worrying that Blackburn Rovers were a rubbish team, they beat Chelsea 2–1.*
>
> *Luv n hugs,*
> *Fran x*

Lee was in the year above at school and intensely passionate about Oasis. I was dating an older man, mature, not like the boys in my year at all. We had an all-consuming teenage love, the sort that makes parents worry about your A levels and hint frequently about birth control. We knew we'd be married at twenty-three, our first child would be called Noel (like in Oasis), our second child would be called Noelle (like in Oasis) and our third child would be called Invisible Ray (I'm not sure why exactly but it probably had something to do with Oasis). We were so in love that he once wished I would die first, because he didn't want me to experience the pain of being without him – thanks Lee. It was going to be Lee to whom I gave my flower, my pearl, my maidenhood. We were going to eat the apple of knowledge together, losing our virginity to each other and living happily ever after.

In preparation of removing our V plates I bought two bumper value-packs of condoms (because let's face it, Lee and I were going to be making love all night long and would probably get through 48 condoms), half with a numbing gel in their tip (because Lee had read that he might not last very long on our first time and a numbing condom might help extend proceedings). It was all planned for our six-month-a-versary at the stroke of midnight. I would enter a new day as a new woman.

Somewhere between the pages of teen magazines and whispers during sleepover parties I'd learnt that there would be pain, my hymen would be brutally punctured and there would be inevitable oceans of blood. That was unless I'd done a lot of horse riding or gymnastics (or gymnastics on horseback, preferably while inserting a tampon). I knew with Lee this wouldn't be the case.

'Does it hurt?' he'd ask (because he was considerate like that), the 1,000 tea lights we'd lit reflected in his eyes. I'd nod bravely, never breaking eye contact for a second, and use the power of our love to sail bravely through into womanhood. Two minutes later the pain would be replaced by . . . something better than pain, although I wasn't really sure what that would be.

My school was located in a borough with one of the highest rates of STDs in London, so our sex education came very much down to watching a nurse put a condom on a purple plastic penis over and over again: 'Put it on. DON'T GET AN AIR BUBBLE IN THE TIP and roll, roll, roll it down the shaft. DROP AND ROLL! DROP AND ROLL!' We learnt not to wear lipstick while having sex as this might break a latex condom, resulting in us contracting all of the STDs displayed vibrantly on the overhead projector (the only time my school ever paid for such vivid colour printing). It was implied that it was a girl's job to know how to put the condom on and at the back of the classroom, we shared tips about how to do this using just your mouth to drive them extra wild. N.B Early experiments showed this technique to be a choking hazard, it would take just one strong inhalation and you've got a condom lodged in your windpipe.

I remember sex education once being left to a substitute Geography teacher who with genuine fear in his eyes, declared, 'BEWARE OF PRE-COME, THE MOST DANGEROUS OF LIQUIDS', which made it hard to concentrate on the different types of destructive lava during exam prep the next lesson.

If I felt ill-equipped, I cannot even imagine being LGBTQIA+ in that classroom. There was not a second's consideration that penis-in-vagina sex might not be the kind we'd be having. Changes are afoot yet sex education always seems to be deprioritised and pushed down the list of essential subjects. Hopefully, by the time you read this book all sex education will be perfect and you'll be thinking, 'what an archaic idea that sex education wasn't thorough and inclusive'. That's happened right?

Things I was taught about in sex education:

- Wet dreams.
- Penis erections.
- The amount of sperm in one ejaculation (20 million to 100 million sperm cells per millilitre of ejaculate and each and every single sperm could get you pregnant).

Things that were not taught:

- That I had a clitoris.
- That I could orgasm.
- That I could enjoy sex.
- That I could say 'no'.
- That consent is more than just saying 'no'.
- That sex was something for me, too.

At sixteen, I could have told you more about photosynthesis and the causes of the Cuban Missile Crisis than about what was between my own legs and how any of it worked. I hadn't considered sex was for me to enjoy at all and any conversations about me 'receiving' went as follows (again, incredibly verbatim).

LEE: Can I lick you out?
ME: What? Like a yoghurt pot?
LEE: I guess?
ME: Why? What's in it for you?
LEE: It's just what we're meant to *do* . . .

ME: Why on earth would you want to *do* that?

Lee shrugs and starts to play Snake on his phone

ME: Ok, but only if I can turn the lights off. You
   mustn't see . . . *it*.

Cue 45 minutes of Lee trying desperately to find my vulva
in the dark. He mostly did not find my vulva, instead
giving me a very soggy upper thigh. I should have helped
him out, but I didn't really know any better.

It would have been useful to know SEX IS FUN AND
ENJOYABLE and that SEX IS FOR YOU TOO and that
YOUR VAGINA IS SELF-CLEANSING and DO WHAT-
EVER YOU WANT WITH YOUR PUBES. Without this
knowledge, the danger is you endure. You are passive. You are done
to. It is fine to consensually be passive, but it should be a choice.

I had absorbed from school corridors that vulvas and vaginas
smelt, were ugly and people were making big sacrifices if they
went down there. This meant you should be grateful if someone deigned to venture there and make it as pleasant and
groomed as possible for them. I'd made the mistake, sat in
Religious Studies, aged fourteen, with my legs open, displaying
my M&S pants and heard jeers of 'close your fish' yelled across
the room. I crossed my legs immediately. They weren't compar-
ing my crotch to a fresh seafood platter caught using sustainably
ethical fishing. This was more the suggestion of an open tin of
dolphin-unfriendly tuna left out in the heat.

Have you ever been shamed for your genitals?

*I used to worry about my labia being too fat, too droopy, too
lopsided. Did it smell too much? Was I too wet, too dry, etc.? One*

guy would like me clean-shaven (so I ignorantly obeyed to please), the next guy would prefer more of a 'landing strip'. 34, f

I'm trans so I have a bizarre relationship with it anyway, but sometimes it can smell and make me so embarrassed. 36, non-binary

I did feel ashamed about it as my inner labia was really long and even used to hurt, so I had a labiaplasty when I was eighteen. 33

Boys at school would always joke about 'minge', 'fishy smells' and 'cabbage/cauliflower'. 22, f

Before I even felt my vagina was broken in sexual ways, I was part of this *leg-crossing, pube-erasing* (I once individually tweezed out every single front-on-visible pube . . . I had too many near misses with bathroom scissors and once removed a layer of skin with a home waxing kit), *vulva-rinsing* club. At thirty not much had changed; I sometimes stopped men going down on me and guided them towards penetrative sex for fear of watching them pick pubes from between their teeth, and watched the clock worrying that they had been down there too long, like a diver nervously watching their oxygen tank.

After some early attempts at foreplay, sixteen-year-old Fran wanted the 'real thing'; she wanted to *make love*. Again, I wish this diary entry wasn't as verbatim as it is.

Dear diary,
I write this not meaning to be funny, but to genuinely express the troubles of a sex life. Me and Lee are very much in love, both think that we really will be together forever in life, want to take

things to the next level . . . five times we have wanted to make love and retained our virginity.

I'm not claiming to be upset by this, if anything it's made me love Lee even more (if that is even possible). I'm sure sex was never meant to be this hard but 5 times it went wrong:

1. *Used a condom with a special 'perform-numbing gel lubricant', got it on (by which I mean the condom not the sex), couldn't get it in because it was painful for me. Numbing agent numbed EVERYTHING for Lee. No sex.*
2. *Got condom on, very painful trying to get it in, no sex.*
3. *Couldn't get condom on (realise we've been putting it on back- to-front and that's why it won't roll down). Had to use second condom, lucky I bought so many. Couldn't get penis in. No sex.*
4. *Got the condom on easy-peasy, some difficult manoeuvring and then so much pain. Couldn't get penis in. It's not important. I love Lee too much to feel disheartened. If anything, I respect him and know more that he is the guy for me. Celibate or not. No big deal, our friendship is too strong for physical cracks to appear.*
5. *Tried to create atmosphere. Made room pretty with candles, flowers and even tidied for sex with Lee . . . pain, no sex.*

Lee and I could only try to have sex on Friday evenings because of homework, so a week would pass and then we'd regroup and try a new tactic . . .

6. *Lee and I mentally prepared. I made a tent in the garden with 2 wooden chairs and a bed sheet, like a romantic canopy. He got a runny nose and sinus pain. No sex.*

7. *Accidentally bled on Lee's sheets, SO embarrassing. Lay frozen on that exact spot all night so he wouldn't see the stain and then remade his entire bed when he went for a shower in the morning. He didn't notice that his sheets were blue and then suddenly white. No sex.*

8. *Used easy-on condoms. Couldn't get it on, it is not 'easy-on' as described. Tried without a condom, pain, no sex.*

Despite my vigorous condom education, putting a condom on an actual living person was not as easy as the sex education nurse had demonstrated. Then even when I got past the hurdle of putting a condom on a penis and tried to have sex, it was as if my vulva had been replaced by a brick wall.

> *Dear diary,*
> *Sex still isn't working. Perhaps my vagina is broken, or doesn't exist, or maybe I'm just not meant to have sex.*

We kept going . . .

9. *Asked Lee to put his penis in unerect and then we could kiss to make it harden inside me. Figured putting his penis inside me soft would mean no pain. But what would happen is he'd come towards me soft, get up to me, his penis would harden, there would be pain, wouldn't go in . . . so he'd retreat, his penis would soften . . . we'd just chill for a bit. Then he'd come back towards me, penis would harden, not go in, pain, etc. etc. No sex. Sort of like a sexy barn dance.*

> *Approach your partner condom in hand*
> *Kiss your partner once or twice*

Get an erection – because kissing is nice
Yeeee haaaa
Penis won't go in, go find another partner to do the
  grapevine with . . .

After six months of trying, Lee and I still hadn't managed to have penetrative sex. My worry about my broken vagina was secondary to my terror that he would leave me for someone with a more accommodating, roomy, welcoming vagina, which at this point my teenage brain thought was everyone with one. I had to prevent Lee leaving me with the only tool I felt I had in my sexual arsenal: blow jobs.

Blow jobs were my apology for not being able to have penetrative sex, each one essentially saying, 'please don't leave me, please don't find someone else, look what my marvellous mouth can do'. I had read a lot of articles about giving the perfect blow job and felt my skills made me an unleavable girlfriend. Lee would never break up with someone who was so expert at keeping one eye on his penis, and one eye making overly intense sexy eye contact, while swivelling (a move teenage magazines called 'The Helter Skelter'). If Lee was disheartened about us not having penetrative sex, I had a blow job ready as compensation. It became a sexual currency. Even if my neck was tired, I was happy that he was happy and that felt like enough.

10. *Lee asked me if I was sure I had a hole. I'm sure there is*
    one, I can put tampons in it, but when it comes to Lee's
    penis it's a big dead end. Lee has asked if it means he is
    really big . . . I have said . . . Sure?

I was taught at school that virginity was a penis entering a vagina. Losing your V plates was like perforating the lid of a yoghurt pot – your hymen was a dairy freshness seal and once opened your value was questionable. The word and concept of virginity just isn't very useful for most people, especially for anyone not having penetrative sex. It was however deeply carved into my teenage self, which is why the grand opening of my Müller Corner had to be perfect.

What did you think losing your virginity would be like and did it meet your expectations? (Feel free to define virginity however you wish.)

Virginity – penetrative sex definition: very underwhelming and was about male pleasure. Virginity – oral definition: amazing. Life-changing.

It came a LOT later than expected, at age 28. As someone who wasn't able to have penetrative sex for the first year of my relationship, I would not define my virginity as the moment my boyfriend put his penis in my vagina.

The first time I had sex without it being painful, it was an enormous relief. In fact, I could barely look past the elation that I could finally fit a whole penis inside of me without crying and therefore didn't even care much for the actual act. I'm trying hard to drop the phrase, 'When I lost my virginity', and instead say, 'When I first had penetrative sex' – as well as finding a new word for 'foreplay' because uh, we need to celebrate that WAY MORE than thinking it's just some sad little 'prequel' sequence. 26, f

Virginity wasn't a helpful word for many of the people I spoke to. It didn't represent their experience of sex at all, and added too many unrealistic expectations.

Being pansexual, I found myself defining virginity in such a way that I 'lost it' twice. The first time was with my first girlfriend. We had no idea what we were doing, but in that we found more pleasure since we had no expectations to live up to. When I lost my virginity in the more 'traditional' sense it felt kind of weird and I didn't get much pleasure from it. 23, f

Losing my virginity for me was absolutely about penetration . . . which was really unpleasant at best! After the 'event'? I was left feeling confused, unsatisfied, embarrassed and then annoyed when he said to me that he didn't think that I was a virgin! 61, f

I haven't lost my virginity but I think it's going to be painful. 21

I wonder now whether if I hadn't defined 'virginity' as this Disneyesque, sword-in-the-stone, coming-of-age style ceremony, would it have been easier? Imagine if I'd been taught then about my own body's capacity for pleasure or even some consent education that was framed positively. I might have been in a very different place fourteen years later when I turned thirty. This diary entry from me at sixteen felt far too familiar.

Dear diary,

Ok I'd never fake anything but sometimes I may emphasise my enthusiasm when he's down there just because it boosts his confidence and I can see how happy it makes him and I don't want us both to feel like total failures.

Today I had my first ever detention, but Lee had one too, both were hungry afterwards, we had Nando's.

I did eventually manage to lose my 'virginity'. The day it happened I proudly wrote about it in my diary, using a special commemorative red gel pen.

Dear diary,
Last night I made love to the most caring, special person I have ever met. It was totally unplanned. Lee and I had sex. We maintained eye contact throughout. Afterwards I insisted he have a cigarette like in the movies and also more than that I wanted to commemorate the event, so I gave him a 2 pence coin to keep with him always, as a sort of war medallion to honour the battle he had valiantly fought against my hymen.

That's what I wrote in my diary anyway. What I didn't write was that it was the hottest sweatiest day of the year, we weren't even really trying to have sex that time but it just sort of happened and his small black cat watched us unflinchingly throughout (perhaps the cat was the charm we'd been missing). In my own personal private diary, I romanticised losing my virginity to myself, unwilling to write down what it was actually like. I thought I would look different afterwards. I hoped I would sound wiser, like I had suddenly gained lots of grown-up knowledge as a card-carrying member of the 'lost my virginity' club. I wondered if other people could tell. Surely other people could tell? Surely, I was glowing?

The complete truth is that after nine months of trying, finally losing my virginity was extremely painful, was over *very* quickly and Lee dumped me the week after. Yep.

* * *

Self-Massage

I am an incredibly anxious human being.

In the 1960s, researchers Masters and Johnson found that stress was at the heart of most sexual dysfunctions and that anxiety and muscle tension massively got in the way of arousal and enjoyment.[14] They developed a technique called Sensate Focus, where couples would touch each other's bodies with curiosity, initially without chasing desire or orgasm. In their studies participants were banned from sexual activity, to increase focus on their own body's responses without pressure or anxiety of performance. With this in mind, I wanted to spend some time on self-massage, not genital focused, not with any goal in mind, but simply touching my body non-sexually.

I'm all for the idea of someone else massaging me. Yes please! Where do I sign up? Pour the oil all over me, light those candles and press play on my favourite panpipe/whale/birdsong album! But doing this for myself? To be honest, I've always felt . . . what's the point?

My moisturising (if it happens at all) is normally practical, brief and without any tenderness. I splash it on, rub it in and run around hastily wafting and blowing on it, avoiding getting my clothes all Nivea-y in the pursuit of glowing skin. When someone else massages me, I love it, so why couldn't I get my head around doing this nice thing for myself? Why couldn't I give my body a nice treat or let it have a little luxury.

I set a timer for twenty minutes, took a moisturiser and slowly, very slowly, and sensually applied this to my body. I had to really focus on the sensations, remind myself to keep breathing and when I found my mind wandering, gently brought it back to my fingertips and how the touch felt. This was another way of practising mindfulness, staying present with my body and breath. I realised that mindfulness can be active (not just sitting cross-legged staring at a raisin) and instead of wanting a quick fix and feeling disappointed that I didn't have one, I really took the time to notice did any body parts feel more? Or less? Or completely the same? I tried not to judge those feelings, just notice them.

At first my mind was racing and my fluttering thoughts were getting in the way of feeling any sensation, but every time I practise I get better at slowing down, feeling more and showing my body some care.

HONEST CONVERSATIONS ABOUT SEX
Sex is up a bit, left a bit, right a bit, ooh it's out again

A: Woman, bisexual, she/her, 28
B: Woman, queer, she/her, 31

A: Talking about sex is super important to me because I'm a sexual health nurse, I know how many people don't talk about sex and how unhappy it makes them.

B: I came out about three years ago, I was the first woman you'd slept with.

A: The first time I had to be like, 'I've never had sex with a lady before'

B: I had an inkling. When I've slept with women, if you're the more dominant one then you are 'the top'. When you are 'the top' it is all about giving pleasure and you sometimes don't get much in return, but in this relationship everyone is getting what they need.

A I'm proud of the fact that we can talk about it, pause halfway and be like, 'No I don't like this, please change that'.

B: We are in hysterics mostly, especially in the early strap-on days . . . when it was my first time using a strap-on.

A: Because you can't feel anything, it was a lot of 'up a bit, left a bit, right a bit, ooh it's out again'.

B: What sex advice would you give?

A: Use more lube, that's my piece of advice to every patient I've ever met, use it on your own, use it with a partner. I used to not use it because I was too embarrassed and without lube it was very painful and uncomfortable.

B: My advice would be to be bossier, say what you want, there are lots of people out there who don't have orgasms because they don't feel like they can tell their partner, whatever gender, what they want. I was that person for years.

A: I think in the past we'd both just had too much shit sex.

B: My sex education at school was anyone who was in a couple went into a room and got spoken to about contraception.

A: They didn't talk about pleasure at all.

B: They don't talk about any other type of sex other than what would get you pregnant and nothing on consent. There are so many types of sex.

A: I think if we stopped talking about what is sex and what isn't sex and trying to define it, it would probably be much easier.

B: The whole concept of virginity as a gay woman is so weird . . . there are so many gay women out there who haven't had sex with a man and so are *technically* virgins. I don't think it's a particularly helpful word.

A: As someone who was *technically* a virgin until they were 19 it would have been a lot easier without the word. One of my friends was like you can't be in your 20s and still be a virgin, so I didn't have a great time the first time.

B: I don't think anyone does.

A: We use sex toys.

B: Please don't say the name that we've called the strap-on.

A: We use a strap-on, also a massage wand thing, occasionally a bullet vibrator.

B: I had a hang-up about using a strap-on, because of my ex, she had a whole feminist thing about how lesbians shouldn't use a strap-on because it's basically a penis, so I was a little 'I don't need a strap-on' but then I realised I was being a bit of an idiot.

A: We picked the least penis-like one, it's purple . . . some of them have balls on the end!

B: I never orgasmed until I had sex with women. I had sex with people because I thought I had to have sex with people, so it took a while to enjoy myself rather than seeing it as a necessary chore.

A: I mean you do still say, 'Is it ok if we don't have sex tonight?'

B: That's because of my fear of lesbian bed death.

A: I didn't know that was a thing, but to be fair I've never been a lesbian before.

B: I think it can happen in all relationships. I think often what people think lesbian sex is, it's often based on porn or some non-existent scissoring thing that isn't a thing. It's unhelpful when you are trying to work out who you are, if you can't even work out what the sex you might be having if you came out would be like. I thought lesbian sex was just like 'strap on and flop about'.

A: I mean, we do flop about quite a bit

4

Being 'That Sort of Girl' & an Abusive Relationship

So, I had turned thirty.

I had recovered from my break-up. Mostly.

I had made myself an online dating profile and I was
  ready to have some fun.

*I'd like to fuck you in the mouth so you can taste yourself on
  my cock*

Come on Skype

Get on Skype

*Can we do a Skype and then I promise I'll never contact you
  again.*

Every morning I woke up to a stream of messages from
  potential suitors, all battling for an audience with my
  heart and my loins.

Come over now and watch Star Wars *porn with me*

Tell me sex things, I'm working and I require distraction.

*Look Frances, why don't you cut to the chase and send me a
  picture of you in your underwear,*

there's only so much small talk I can manage.

And even though I wasn't looking for anything serious, I also wasn't prepared for the tone of many of the *sweet nothings* I was sent.

Want ths dick deep in ur throat?

Anal only though. No kissing. They're my rules.

You are going to need an ice pack.

My selection process was overseen by my friend Laura. Over the weeks since I turned thirty, she had steadily gripped her wine glass more and more tightly, as I read to her the types of replies I got to my standard opening lines on dating apps.

Sex now Fran, or unmatch me. Don't waste my time frigid slut.

Laura and her husband would laugh, wince and grimace, like my dating life was a gripping but titillating new BBC drama that they couldn't look away from. This was a role I seemed to have slipped into, the relationship jester, providing married friends with thrills, a gladiator fighting wildly for the benefit of the dating arena emperor.

Between the demands for immediate sex, I had landed on someone I liked the look of. He seemed friendly, lived nearby and had no photographs of himself holding endangered animals or protesting too much that the children he was cuddling weren't his. Perfect. After a week of chatting online, I had arranged to meet him at a pub conveniently equidistant to both of our houses, which he had told me had a good selection of crisps. My remit was clear, I was going to go out with this man and if I fancied him and the mood was right, we were going to have sex and I was going to follow my new rules. If we wanted to see each other again, sure, great, but also, I was going to be just fine walking into the sunset post-sex, never to see each other again.

'I've got a good feeling about him,' said Laura, as we drank a glass of wine in her kitchen ahead of my date that evening. Her husband washed the dishes calmly, as Laura's thumbs glided rapidly over photos of my date.

'He's got the eyes of an attentive lover, strong brows and really nice teeth.'

Laura and I have been friends since school, and I tell her mostly everything, but I had never been brave enough to share the whole truth about my experience with sex. This was because our sex lives couldn't have been more different. Laura had told me that her and her husband of ten years make love at least three times every week, Monday, Wednesday and Sunday (the Sunday sex is mostly mid-morning, before an Earl Grey tea and a browse through the newspapers in bed) and only ever refer to it as making love. She had told me that they both 'achieve climax' every single time, often simultane-ously. When she talked about bad sex, it was falling over when having adventurous lovemaking in the shower and neighbours knocking on their walls because their lovemaking was making their lampshade wobble. She made her sex life sound like it was straight out of a movie, all soft focus, low lighting and no sweat. There was no pain, no disappointment, no tears and no pretending.

Laura's husband stopped washing up for a moment and peered over her shoulder. 'The best thing to do is *not* sleep with him tonight Fran,' he said. 'Leave him wanting more. Else he will think you are *that sort of girl* Fran . . . and you aren't *that sort of girl* Fran.'

'There's nothing wrong with casual sex,' I replied. 'It's empowering and exciting. It's important, to recognise your own sexual wants, fulfill them, without the outdated clingy trappings of relationships. Not like your relationship of course, your relationship is obviously not outdated or clingy or in any way trapping.'

I'd said these words in defence of casual sex, but felt the sting of the phrase 'that sort of girl'. Maybe from tiny slurs planted at school, whispers about girls who would 'go with anyone', slut-shaming graffiti written on tables, boys being high-fived for sleeping with a girl, while girls were labelled as easy, sluts, hoes, frigid and cock teases indiscriminately. Whatever sexual decisions we made it never felt like anyone was getting it right. As an adult I felt I was ridiculously still playing those games, attempting to find the perfect balance between not sleeping with someone so fast that they thought I had a revolving door vagina, or so late that they might lose interest. These ideas should have stayed and died in the playground.

Laura's husband chuckled as he rinsed a colander. 'Just don't give it away too easily, yeah? Or they'll lose respect for you and you deserve respect, you aren't like *that.*'

Laura smiled at me apologetically.

Like *that*? Like what? What exactly was it I was giving away?

I knew that the only person who should be allowed to have an opinion on my sex life was me, but his words had still prickled me. I think truthfully I always hoped that any casual sex I might have might turn into a fully committed relationship. So, I guess my casual sex had always been more smart-casual, than casual–casual.

Research suggests that women have better sex in committed relationships.[15] There's also been some research into sexual regret, which found that women regret having casual sex more than men do: men regret not having more casual sex.[16] Look a little sideways of these facts and you will find studies that suggest that yes, this is true, but if the sex is good then women are far less likely to regret it and women who feel positively and really want to have casual sex are much more likely to have higher orgasmic function and sexual satisfaction from it.[17] So, feeling positively about casual sex (rather than the shame, anxiety and worry) makes it more likely for it to be an enjoyable experience. Not a huge surprise there.

As I left Laura's house for my date, she kissed me on the cheek. 'Be safe. Have fun. And don't listen to him, if you want to sleep with your date you go for it, there's no such thing as *that sort of girl.*'

I nodded, squeezed her hand and walked the half-hour to the pub with a good selection of crisps. The phrase 'that sort of girl' had burrowed under my skin. I gave myself a pep talk. It didn't matter what Laura's husband thought, or anyone else for that matter, I was going to enjoy myself, like the sexually liberated woman I was.

One of the first questions my prospective wooer asked me once we'd both sat down, was how many men I'd slept with. Yeah, I thought it was an odd opening question too – and I didn't even think to ask him the same question back. But I answered – 'about fifteen'.

'Fifty?!' (I guess I am a bit of a mumbler).

He put his pint down heavily. Fifty was excessive, fifty was legions of men, basically most of the global population. He joked that he probably knew some of them and I found myself hurriedly correcting him. Fifteen, it was *only* fifteen, thirty-five shagging partners closer to virginity. He laughed and said that sounded more 'accurate', although it was 'still more than a whole football team'. Perhaps this judgmental banter meant he was heavily into me, perhaps we'd laugh at this mumbling mix-up on our wedding day. Except for there wouldn't be a wedding day, I had to keep reminding myself I was just there for the most casual of casual sex experiences.

'Good to know you're not like *that*. Fifty, imagine,' he added.

A person who connects someone's number of sexual partners with their worth should be avoided at all costs. What I should have done was place my own pint glass down heavily, perhaps knocked it over in his lap, left the bar and not given him a second thought. Instead I ended up having sex with him.

I was sure we must both be thinking that this date was going terribly, watching the clock, wondering how early it was polite enough to leave. When he asked me if I wanted another pint, I should have said no.

'Yes,' I found myself saying, 'yes, yes please.'

He was about to head off for the bar, when he turned and kissed me so hard and so unexpectedly that I almost fell off my stool.

I repeat, with hindsight, it is clear that I should not have had sex with this person. I should have walked away from this one immediately.

I'd like to be able to explain exactly why I did have sex with him, but I can't. I can only make half-hearted guesses that maybe I felt oddly flattered that he liked me, honoured that he had been brave, taken a chance and kissed me and perhaps that should be rewarded with my time, right? That was passionate, right? Courageous? Bold? Kissing someone who hasn't shown any interest in kissing you was romantic, right? I'd seen that romcom.

Half an hour later we were at his house kissing on his bed.

'Wait' I said. Despite the surprise kissing I was still determined for the sexual experience to be one in which I was confident and in control. This meant for me starting to ask for the things I wanted and needed to have better sex. Number one on my list was using lube.

'I'd like to use some lube,' I said. His face fell.

'I've got some with me,' I continued, reassuring him, wanting to ease his mind that he didn't have to run out to the Co-op to get some. He looked repulsed.

'You brought lube with you? Bit presumptuous. You thought you were definitely getting some?' He was smiling but it wasn't the kindest of smiles.

Perhaps, I thought, perhaps he'd had a bad experience with lube in the past. There's a lot of flavoured, tingly, sensation enhancing, pH-changing lubes that just don't agree with everyone's genitals.

'It's organic,' I added.

'I'll just *make* you wet,' he said. 'You won't *need* lube with me. I'm as organic as it comes.'

I got the lube out of my bag ready, just in case. In the throes of passion, I presumed he would probably be more open to it.

'Seriously, you aren't going to need that, I know what I'm doing.'

I realised this probably wasn't the time for me to launch into an explanation about how a lot of the time the amount a person's vagina becomes lubricated has very little to do with how turned on they are feeling in their brain and body. It's probably not the moment to say, 'There's this thing called arousal non-concordance, it means you could be in the most arousing of situations with all your turn on needs met and not feel genitally aroused at all.[18] It can also mean you are shopping in Lidl, picking up a jar of peanut butter, and suddenly you're very wet, which probably doesn't mean you want to have intercourse with a crushed peanut-based spread'. It wasn't the time, but also in all honesty, I didn't know those things yet. I thought the body was simple: Turned On = lubricated, Turned Off = dry, Fran = broken.

I felt so small and naïve in that moment, sat there holding my organic lube (honestly, look at the back of some tubes of lube, you don't want to be putting a lot of those chemicals on your vulva). I had everything I wanted to ask for lined up in my head, but I just couldn't bring myself to say it. I told myself that asking for things would get easier, that next time I would be more assertive. The next time I had sex I would get it more right.

The following happened:

The sex was bare minimum.

He went straight for penetration. No build-up.

I was incredibly dry.

He rolled his eyes when I asked for foreplay.

He thrusted his fingers in and out of my vagina for about half a minute, his nod to foreplay.

He was inside me far before I was ready.

It was painful but I said nothing.

I lifted my hips to make it be over quicker.

I made some small noises of enjoyment to speed him along. I was less vociferous than I would be with someone I love, because, well, I cared less.

I asked if I could go on top, he didn't reply.

It was rough, leaving marks on my skin.

Immediately after ejaculating, he fell asleep.

As he snored, I silently and secretly spooned him as hard I could. I was trying to squeeze things into feeling a bit normal.

In hindsight it is clear, I should not have had sex with this man. I should have just left as soon as I realised I wasn't enjoying the date. Or when he kissed me forcefully out of nowhere. Or when he sneered at me for asking for lube. Or first thing the next morning. Yes, those are definitely points at which I should have left.

'How are things going with the man?' Laura asked over a cup of tea several weeks later. 'You've been seeing him a lot. Must be going well? Has it turned into something more serious?'

'Oh, you know, really . . . great, just really good,' I replied, rolling my eyes, hoping that would explain everything and nothing.

'You see,' her husband said triumphantly. 'Isn't this better than just bed hopping?'

I'd love to say I took control of my sexual destiny the next week. Or the week after, or even the month after.

I actually saw him again, and again and again, over many months.

I know. I know.

I kept seeing him, I didn't seem able to stop.

I told myself that even one nice-ish experience with him would make me feel like I hadn't wasted my time or been treated badly. I told myself that if I kept going back, I could undo how degraded I felt and make things right and fresh. I found myself wanting to make it feel like a solid relationship, because then there would be a reason I kept going back, then there would be something solid to fix. One Friday evening, we were watching a documentary about gambling. It spoke about sunk cost fallacy, where a gambler will keep playing at the table, far beyond the point at which they should have left the casino, just to try and desperately grasp some of their losses back. I looked at the man next to me and realised, 'That's me. I am a sunk cost fallacy'. I knew I should walk away, but like a gambler on a losing streak, I was sure I could make it right. I was sure I could still win something back.

'I don't like it when you tell me what to do in bed,' he said, one time after having sex. 'It makes me feel like you don't trust my ability. It also ruins the surprise . . . like, where's the spontaneity if you know what I'm going to do next?' We argued in bed about vocal consent. I thought it might be sexy to hear what each other wants. He disagreed. He believed passion came from two people instinctively working things out in the moment, responding to each other's bodies and that words had no place between the sheets. The conversation took away my words entirely.

I know now that this was a deeply unhealthy situation to have found myself in. I would advise anyone who is in a relationship that is making them unhappy to seek support to get out of it. It isn't always easy to just walk away. I didn't feel like I could talk to anyone about it, because I was embarrassed, I felt like I should have known better. I also didn't think it was 'bad enough' to need help, but this isn't true. I had become so passive in this that I was letting my body be used for someone else's pleasure, with no consideration for my own wellbeing and mental health.

One particular day I noticed at the last minute that he wasn't wearing a condom. I stopped him immediately and sprang out of bed. He rolled his eyes and rolled onto his front simultaneously, saying, 'We've been dating for long enough now to not use condoms. Don't you trust me?'

I had heard of people using all kinds of excuses to not wear condoms: 'I'm too big', 'It ruins the moment', 'I can't feel and enjoy the sex properly when I'm wearing one'. But this was the first time it had happened to me.

'It'll be more fun without a condom,' he continued. 'Don't you want us to have fun? You always have to make everything so serious. I thought you were fun.'

I sat there thinking about fun and realising that actually I wasn't having that much fun at all. I looked at my body, which was quite bruised from all the sex the way he liked it.

'You are the first person who I've been with who *insists* on always using a condom,' he added. I didn't want to be boring; I didn't want to be not fun.

'Is it because you are sleeping around? Is that why you insist on us using them?'

'I'm not sleeping around.'

'Well then, what's the problem Fran? Help me trust you.'

Part of me wanted to just get back under the covers with him to make this all go away. There was however a small but persistent voice in my head that knew this was sexual coercion, that I was being pressured and emotionally manipulated into having sex that I did not want.

It took this exchange for me to wonder how a one-night experiment at casual sex had turned into something that was so unhealthy and was still lingering months later.

So I left, got in a taxi and travelled to Laura's house, where she made a pot of tea, sent her husband out of the house and ran me a hot bath.

I wondered if she knew. I wasn't quite ready to tell her everything.

'I'm finding sex hard. Not good. Not enjoying it' I said.

She nodded sympathetically. I carried on.

'I've actually always found it really hard, ever since I was sixteen.'

I told her about trying to lose my virginity with Lee, about eventually managing penetrative sex but still finding it painful, about faking enjoyment to get it over more quickly and about sometimes just not feeling like I want sex at all because of dreading the fact that it's going to hurt.

For a moment I wished I hadn't said anything, as we sat in silence for a comfortably uncomfortable minute. I was worried she'd be upset or feel betrayed that I'd not shared any of this with her before.

'I finish myself off,' she said. 'Once he's finished finishing. Once he's asleep mostly.'

'I thought you came every time?'

'I do, mostly, but sometimes, it's me who does the last push.'

'Does he know?' I asked. She shook her head.

She carried on, 'I also know I should be ok with having sex on my period but I'm just not and I think that maybe makes me a bad feminist but I just can't stop thinking about the white sheets and the mess. It's a really hard mess to wash out.' She paused. 'And I get really bad thrush. So bad, I should go to the doctors about it but I keep putting it off, because I'm worried they'll tell me off for not going sooner.'

We sat in the bathroom looking at each other.

'Sorry, that's quite a lot isn't it, I just wanted you to know, you aren't on your own.'

I decided I couldn't face telling her that day about the relationship; I hadn't quite worked it out for myself at that point. Embarrassed and ashamed for not being able to leave it sooner and wrongly worried that she would judge me, I kept silent. I did tell her about it much later and she recommended that I go and speak about it with someone professional and gently suggested that what I had considered an unhappy relationship had actually been an abusive one. She told me much, much later that she had known for a while that something wasn't right, but hadn't known how to help. But on that day with me in the bath and her perched on the toilet seat, as we sat there sharing some smaller sexual secrets, she was determined to help me and so without saying another word, she got out her laptop and together we started looking for a solution.

We google . . .

Sex is painful

Why can't I orgasm?

Is my vagina broken?

Is my vagina haunted?

There was an acronym that kept popping up, bracketing together difficulty orgasming, pain during sex and low libido: FSD: Female Sexual Dysfunction. A label. A diagnosis even, maybe? It took into account that my three areas of sexual difficulty impacted each other. Of course it would be harder to orgasm if sex was painful; of course sex might be painful if I wasn't aroused enough; of course it might be harder to want sex if my experiences so far had been disappointing and painful. What a sexy Venn diagram that would be!

83

FSD. It wasn't the sexiest sounding name, but it resonated with me, with the fact that my painful sex didn't seem to fit into any one box, with the fact that my body didn't feel like it was working, with the fact that my brain often felt like it lived on a different continent to my vagina.

Laura put her hand on mine, 'If sex hurts you should go to the doctor, Fran, I know that's rich coming from me . . . because of the thrush . . . but I don't think sex should hurt.'

* * *

Lubricant

It took me a long time after my experiences with this man to feel comfortable about using and asking to use lube during sex. Bringing it on dates had already felt like a confession that my body wasn't always the natural spring/ powerful erupting geyser I wanted it to be or felt it *should* be. After the belittling remarks he had made about me wanting to use lubricant, I'd felt even less positive about it. I needed to build my confidence and so decided to speak to a connoisseur of vaginal lubricants to help me select one that worked for me. Luckily, I had met a lady who puts the 'can' in lubricant, the person who is affectionately revered as The Lady of the Lube, Lavinia Winch. She worked for YES The Organic Intimacy Company.

Lavinia was married in 1978 and had her first baby two years later with a natural delivery, but like many others had an episiotomy (a cut made between the anus and the vagina during childbirth to widen the opening of the vagina – around 1 in 7 deliveries in England involve an episiotomy).[19] When she went back to having sex, at first it was very uncomfortable due to dryness caused by breastfeeding and scar tissue from the procedure.

'In those days, KY was the only lube available from the chemist and so that was our "go to" product. After sex I would get sore, irritated, itchy and uncomfortable around the vagina and the vulva, but I thought it was thrush and often self-treated with anti-thrush medication.' Doctors also told her that she had thrush and a vulval dermatologist prescribed steroid cream for eczema.

'We'd use the cream, but it never cleared up properly and this discomfort went on for thirty years because I was still using standard lubes. It turns out that doctors don't know everything about vaginal and vulval health and sometimes we need to listen to our own bodies. Finally, in 2009 when I started working for The YES YES Company, I began using an organic plant-oil lube and all my vulval issues went away.'

Lavinia is a strong believer that lubricant should be fun, pleasurable and can be used with a partner, for masturbation and with sex toys.

'I think maybe there has been a belief that if you are not wet enough, you have failed or your partner may feel blame for not managing to sufficiently arouse you. There are many reasons why you may not lubricate naturally: during pregnancy, while breastfeeding, after cancer treatment, during times of stress and anxiety, when taking anti-depressants or medication for colds and flu (decongestants). There should be no shame in using lube at any stage of your life and there is absolutely no doubt that this issue of painful sex due to vaginal dryness or other gynaecological conditions can break up relationships.'

Her tips for choosing a good lubricant are:

- Anything you put in the vagina should match vaginal pH of between 3.8 and 4.5. These numbers should be on the packaging, the product or in the instructions. If they aren't, don't buy it! This acidic environment helps to prevent bacteria from thriving which otherwise may lead to Thrush, Bacterial Vaginosis and Urinary Tract Infections.
- It's best to avoid lubricants containing glycerine as this is a sugar product and can feed *candida albicans*, causing Thrush.
- The anus has a different pH. If you put an acidic lube in the anus it might sting; it should be around about pH 7 to match the anus, so look for products that are specifically designed for anal sex.
- If you are using additional lube with condoms, it must be water-based as oil-based lube can damage latex condoms.

'It's so important that we talk about these things, so people don't feel alone and embarrassed. Everyone has the right to be able to enjoy a full and active sex life. Lube is not only helpful for alleviating medical conditions, but it can also add sensitivity, pleasure and enhancement of sensation for everyone.'

Lavinia talks about using lube like it's as obvious as wearing a good sunscreen. Speaking to her reassured me that using it shouldn't be embarrassing, as it can decrease anxiety about pain and friction and increase pleasure during all kinds of sex.

Also, I find lubricant is a good litmus test for sexual partners. If someone reacts badly to you reaching for the lube, or isn't willing to at least have a conversation about using it, they are unlikely to be the most attentive or considerate of lovers . . . maybe best avoid.

HONEST CONVERSATIONS ABOUT SEX
Sex changes all the time when you are pregnant

Woman, heterosexual, she/her, 33

I'm a midwife and I had imagined that sex wouldn't really change very much when I was pregnant, if anything I thought I would feel hornier. The first six weeks were fine and then my sex drive disappeared completely, like I have never known it in my entire life before. I didn't realise prior to this how integral to my identity as an adult woman my sex drive was. And to have it removed, no desire at all! Not even that sort of tired, 'Maybe I could rustle up some sex?' desire. I'd been prepared for sickness, and I'd been prepared for tiredness, but I hadn't been prepared for this complete lack of sex drive. There were a few times when I thought I'll try and have sex and I discovered that in the meantime my body had completely changed, my vagina felt completely different. I was and continue to be incredibly sensitive to touch . . . any touch now has to be as light as a feather. My husband and I have been together for a while, he knows what I like, I know what he likes and all of a sudden, things that had always worked didn't work.

My sex drive didn't come back with any significance until I was maybe sixteen weeks pregnant. It was like a switch being turned back on, I was like 'Hold on, I actually have the horn'. But then my body had changed *again* and it all felt different *again*. My orgasms have completely changed, which I'm sure is really amusing for the neighbours, because now I can't stop laughing when I have an orgasm and I've twice burst into tears, and I'm not a crier. It's all change down there all the time, it has come . . . haha come . . . as quite a surprise.

I think people might think that pregnant women are super horny all the time, but that's the only side of things anyone is willing to share or talk about. I don't think I've ever heard anyone talk about how they've gone off sex during pregnancy . . . maybe only when they are at the very, very end when they can't move for baby. I heard a lot from women that their partners don't want to have sex because they are worried their penis will hit the baby's head. It's not . . . it won't . . . it's not going to.

I don't think the responsibility of sexual welfare of a pregnant woman falls to anyone, we talk about contraception, but there's no writ that says the midwife, the health visitor or the GP has to talk or ask about sex ever again. A lot of people need to be referred to a specialist physio after birth but they don't get sent there.

When my sex drive was gone, I was worried that was just it now, that I was just going to be a vessel for this baby, just a mum, and being a mum isn't seen as very sexy. Am I going to be a MILF? I'm not even feeling particularly sexual with myself at the minute, there's just been so much changing but I don't see masturbating as being far off. A friend told me that she has never masturbated as much as she did at the end of her pregnancy in her entire life . . . so we will wait and see what happens with that.

5

The Doctor & The Magic Penis

'Do you want to come . . . upstairs?' My friend was leaning in the doorway, silhouetting himself, like someone who has practised being sexy; he blew his fringe up and looked directly into my eyes. We'd been friends for a while, but there had never been any frisson there. This felt clunky, clumsy and out of nowhere.

'I'm alright thanks,' I said, replying very quickly, 'but thank you . . . thanks. That's a really lovely, *lovely*, nice, kind, nice, *nice* offer. Thank you.' I stood up and immediately asked, 'Shall I put the kettle on?'

Five minutes earlier I'd been venting at this same friend, furious as I sat on one of his snow-white sofas. I saw his brow raise every time I gestured too much with my hands, wine sloshing in glass. I had decided to take Laura's advice and had just visited the doctor to see if there was anything medically wrong with my vagina.

'I really thought that the doctor might be able to help,' I said. 'Did you know that the whole human genome was mapped before anyone did a detailed ultrasound of the clitoris and the clitoris isn't even in a lot of anatomy books, and in the seventeenth century people thought that the clitoris was a birth defect, they thought the clitoris was a tiny penis that women grew if they touched themselves too much and . . .'

I stopped for breath, still fuming but noticing that my friend was staring incredibly shyly into his tea.

'Sorry, is it ok that I tell you this?' I asked, 'I know it's a bit . . . much. A lot. I really had thought going to the Doctor's might help.'

It also wasn't the first time I'd been.

Somewhere between the fumbling Friday night virginity losing attempts and unhelpful sex education lessons, 16-year-old Fran had also plucked up the courage to make an appointment with her doctor to ask them for help with her broken vagina. She'd explained that it felt like there was a door stopping her boyfriend's penis from entering and no matter what she did they couldn't get him in. The response from the doctor was mid-examination:

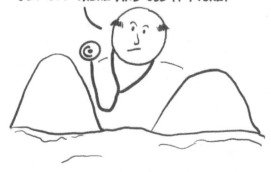

Alongside this was a reassurance that, 'Pain is to be expected when losing your virginity, keep at it and it will get easier.'

The idea that losing your virginity will definitely hurt is hopefully something that is dwindling into myth. It *can* be uncomfortable the first time you have penetrative sex, it will hurt for some people, but generally if you are relaxed and lubricated, pain is not a foregone conclusion. The more we are told that it will be painful, the more likely we are to tense up and anticipate pain, meaning the chances of it hurting are much more likely. The pain I was experiencing at sixteen was put down to my youth and inexperience by my doctor, and I was essentially told to soldier bravely on. I was also handed an overflowing bag of condoms and information about the contraceptive pill, which at the time felt like really rubbing it in my face that I couldn't have sex . . . How did they think I was I going to get pregnant if I couldn't even have sex?

Over the years I had returned to the doctor multiple times . . .

- At nineteen I was told to, 'See if I could get hold of some erotic fiction', because that would sort the problem out.
- At twenty-one to 'Have a glass of wine to loosen up a bit'.
- At twenty-four to, 'Just pop some Savlon on the problem area'.
- And at twenty-six, reassured that 'Things will be better once you have children. Birth creates more space'.

I'd felt dismissed and unheard every single time. At thirty, I was hopeful that medical science might have made some advancements and perhaps with bigger and louder conversations about female pleasure happening, it might be more likely I'd be listened to.

Let me set the scene.

I'd over-thought absolutely every detail to make sure that I didn't panic, get flustered, panic, stutter over my words, PANIC or worse say nothing at all. I was wearing clothes that oozed *grown-up, mature woman, who is comfortable and familiar with her body* (dungarees) and female power anthems were blaring in my headphones (Shakira would never have a problem saying vagina to a doctor). This was the year that a doctor would listen to me and together we'd fix this problem once and for all. On my journey there, I practised the sentence I was going to say over and over, so it was deeply embedded in my muscle memory.

'Hello my name is Fran and I'm here to fix my broken vagina.'

'Hi, Ms Bushe here, I'm here to fix my vag.'

'Good morrow to you fine medics, I am Frances Bushe and I'm here about ye olde vagina!'

Feeling like a confident powerful woman, I swooshed my hair in slow motion as I entered the crowded surgery and signed in. There had been a big emergency that morning, which meant doctors were running late and patients were fidgety and uneasy. It gave me a lot of time to overthink everything even further.

MY BRAIN: What words should I use? I probably shouldn't call it just 'sex'. I should call it: *full penetrative sex*. Or Intercourse. Coitus? Slap and tickle? Bonking? Banging? Making love? Making whoopie? Making the beast with two backs? Should I call it libido or sex drive? Should I let them know the true extent of the googling I've already done? Will my vulva be sweaty from all the power walking I've

done en route? Should I go and splash down my
vulva in the downstairs patient toilet? I don't want
to miss my appointment because I'm too busy
splashing!

Everyone else in the waiting room had visible or audible signs
of illness: broken arms, stitches, spluttering coughs. I felt they
must all be looking at me wondering what on earth was wrong
with me.

MY BRAIN: Maybe I should leave? I'm not ill or sick,
so I shouldn't waste a doctor's time. Someone could
be dying in the waiting room while I'm complaining
about not having a good time between the sheets. I
should cancel my appointment and give space to
people who are really unwell, I'm not *really* unwell, I
just want one little thing to be a little bit better. It's
nothing major!

DR: Sorry for the wait, there's been an emergency this
morning. What can I do for you?

ME: I'm here about not enjoying . . . sex. I find it painful. It's not a medical emergency. I don't think
anyone's ever died from not having sex. Has anyone
ever died from not having sex?

DR: No.

ME: Right. The last time I came I was twenty-four . . .
not *came* sexually you understand, came to the doctor
about this specific problem, and now I'm thirty and
I'd like to fix sex.

(I did a little buck-up 'yeehaa' gesture here. I think it's because I wanted the doctor to have a nice time doctoring me.)

ME: I'm not enjoying sex.

DR: What were you hoping we could do about it?

ME: Well, I would really like to enjoy sex.

DR: How does your partner feel about all of this?

ME: Oh, well I'm actually single right now, so I'm dating a bit but—

DR: Must be hard for him, let's see if we can book you in for couple's psychosexual therapy.

ME: Right. So. It might be a little bit intense to say 'Do you want to have sex . . . *therapy* with me' on a second date. We were just going to go to Pizza Express.

DR: Perhaps you should schedule an appointment when you have a more regular, *committed* partner.

ME: And until then?

DR: Have you ever heard of masturbation?

ME: Yes. Definitely heard of it.

DR: Have you had your babies yet?

ME: No, no babies . . .

DR: What about just not having sex?

ME: I'd like to have sex . . .

DR: There are a group of people who would be very happy just not having sex. Especially if you aren't *trying* for babies.

ME: I'd like to have sex.

DR: Any anxiety? Depression? Low mood?

ME: I do suffer from being anxious. A lot.

DR: I see. Well. There we go.
ME: I googled something called FSD?
DR: Ah, Dr Google.

We sat in silence. The appointment was clearly over from his perspective but neither of us made a move. Surely, he needed to examine me? Or book me in for some tests? Or ask more questions? Eventually I stood up slowly to leave the room, hoping he would stop me, and as I turned to leave he said . . .

'Good Luck!'

Good luck?

GOOD LUCK?

'Good luck' isn't something you say to someone who's come to you for help.

'Good luck' felt like I was completely on my own.

I left the doctor's surgery, furiously grumbling well-researched facts I wish I'd thought to say in the moment, like, 'This is unfair! There are currently twenty-six FDA medically approved solutions for similar disorders in men, who ALREADY orgasm three times as much as straight cisgender women do during sex and it's not a competition (imagine if it was?! So much clean-up) but how is that fair?'

And,

'Viagra was made available over the counter WITHOUT PRESCRIPTION in the UK in 2017 and is advertised on enormous posters in pharmacy windows and on the underground, but there is nothing in the UK for people with vaginas, nothing!'

And,

'We didn't know the clitoris's full structure until 1998. 1998!!?! Why are vulvas so ignored? What about vaginas?'

Underneath this rage, I felt terrible for wasting NHS time, like an idiot for thinking my novelty complaint was a problem, and embarrassed that I had asked a stranger (albeit a medical one) for sex to be enjoyable. I'd made my way straight to my friend's house, ready to vent and probably have a little cry.

I think doctors are incredible. I am proud of the NHS and the amazing work it does. I have had fantastic doctors who treated my childhood asthma, my teenage epilepsy and my adulthood anxiety with professionalism and compassion. But among the people I spoke to, there was a feeling that the quality of care changed when it was something related to sex or reproductive organs.

Has a doctor ever made you feel bad or embarrassed for asking questions about your genitals/reproductive system?

I once asked a nurse about vaginal discharge and she literally screwed her face up and then laughed. 24, f

I had a professional medical doctor tell me I should shave my pubic hair (with embarrassed laughter).

I went to a doctor as I could not come. He had no idea what to say . . . eventually, floundering, he answered, 'Try for yourself?' 39, f

There were stories of embarrassment (on both sides), judgement and often a lack of sensitivity. I was going to include three or four examples here, but as I started asking questions, a far larger more painful problem emerged, an unwillingness to prioritise female sexual problems and a negation of their pleasure . . .

Several doctors told me the pain I was feeling was 'impossible' or 'all in my head'. I was often misdiagnosed. and when treatments didn't work, that some women just have to 'live with the pain'. 25, f

I was dismissed by at least 4 GP's while trying to find out about vaginismus and was only officially diagnosed when I was 27. Some advice I was given was to 'just relax', 'to think about whether I was really attracted to my partner or not' and that 'you're just not ready' – the last one [when] I was 25 years old. 31, f

Mostly they don't know what to do with me, and my issue of painful sex has still not been fully resolved. I've seen five GPs (some examined me, some didn't bother) a nurse, a gynae, a surgeon, two physios and a physio student. More medical professionals have seen my vag than sexual partners. 28

Post-birth was also a very sexually reductive time for people with vaginas. Once you've had a baby your right to sexual pleasure seems secondary to being seen as a mother.

Women in this country are given little to no support after birth. In other countries, women are offered physio for their pelvic muscles and a proper check. Since I had no cuts or tears with either of my children, not a single doctor, midwife or health visitor checked to see if I was ok there. Once my baby was born, the pad went on and no one even asked. I think this is very wrong.

He had a very large head, as all the doctors and nurses liked to tell me — I was well aware of that, thanks! I don't think I was prepared for how much long-term damage childbirth could do. Penetration was painful or uncomfortable for around a year afterwards. I never got checked out properly though, I don't know why. Perhaps I thought it wasn't really a big illness or that important, after all it was only painful or uncomfortable for those minutes and it wasn't like I was walking around in agony. 38, f

I had an episiotomy during the birth of my daughter and the healing process was long and painful. Medical advice was basically 'give it time'. My (otherwise great) GP even offered to give me a doctor's note to 'get me out of sex' for a year. I was too tired and sore to say anything at the time. 40, f

It is not just during sex that vaginal pain can be a problem. Many people I spoke to had experienced upsetting cervical smears.

I was left with trauma after my first smear test, aged 25. I had never had sex and never been able to use tampons, which I told the nurse. However, she clearly didn't listen and used a normal-sized speculum as routine, it was excruciatingly painful and the trauma was caused when I asked her to stop and she didn't.

I'm rather small internally and always tell them so, but they insisted on using equipment that was too big for me. When I cried out in pain, instead of being apologetic or sympathetic, I'd have to endure comments such as 'that's odd, it shouldn't hurt . . .' or, 'Hmm, people don't usually find this

uncomfortable, try to relax . . .' This subliminally made me feel
somehow abnormal or 'to blame' for being different.

I attempted a couple of very painful smear tests, unsuccessfully.
The nurse laughed and said, 'how do you expect to push a baby
out (if I can't even cope with a speculum)?' She probably meant
no harm but I apologised and cried in the toilet. 37, f

Currently cervical screening is at a twenty-year low, with
around one in three women aged twenty-five to sixty-four not
having a smear test every three years (the NHS recommended
time frame).[20] There are things that can be done to help smear
tests be more comfortable and less intimidating:

- Make sure the speculum is the right size for you; it is
  definitely not one size fits all. Fun fact, my vagina is
  extra-long and so the nurse always has to get a longer
  speculum (I used to be weirdly shy to say this as it felt
  brazenly boastful, but now know it saves time just to say
  it upfront).
- You can request a double appointment so the time
  doesn't feel pressurised.
- Ask for a small amount of lubricant to be used on the
  speculum.

The design of the speculum hasn't changed drastically in
150 years and was not designed with vaginal comfort in mind.
Its inventor wrote in his autobiography, 'If there was anything
I hated, it was investigating the organs of the female pelvis',
which didn't really bode well for someone who is often hailed
as the father of American gynaecology.[21] He conducted

surgical experiments on slave women, winning awards for his work, which was often performed in front of a crowd of male doctors, without pain relief. The speculum is now an essential tool in saving people with vaginas lives, but it's development and early use, like so much of 'women's medicine' is overshadowed with a lack of humanity, racism and an abuse of power.

These were just a small selection of the experiences that were shared with me. There were many more. Examples of people being brave enough to ask questions but being made to feel their concerns weren't valid and that their pain and pleasure wasn't important.

Some of it may be my fault, I was too reticent fighting my corner. Not clear enough in my own mind that the problem was real. I should have trusted my instincts and my own knowledge of my body to really insist something was wrong. 46, f

This last one particularly resonated with me. No one should have to 'really insist' there is something wrong with them. We know our bodies better than anyone. Reading these accounts, it felt like people had been gaslit, told that nothing was wrong, even though they could see and feel their symptoms. I had left my own appointment feeling stuck somewhere between wondering if I should have been more demanding and feeling like I shouldn't have gone at all.

If you suspect something is wrong, please, please, please do go to your doctor. I worry that people hearing these stories might be deterred from seeking help, but it is still so important to get any pain, bleeding, discomfort or any changes checked. There are well-informed GPs and specialist clinics out there and you absolutely always have the right to a second opinion. What needs to change is better training for medical practitioners with sexual and vaginal concerns. Medical professionals and trainees I spoke to said . . .

Medically you do have a right to not be in pain, but no right to enjoyment.

Sexual and reproductive health are such a small part of the medical curriculum.

I think it's a lack of training and time. GPs have no formal training on this and Female Sexual Dysfunction isn't funded by the NHS.

I'm not sure where someone would refer you to.

It's hard to untangle sex from vaginas, so sometimes GPs do get embarrassed and worried about saying something sexual.

It would be several years before I met people who were supportive, helpful and convinced me that my experience wasn't all in my head. I want to introduce you to a few of these people, to reassure you that there are kind experts out there, they can be tricky to find, but when you do, it can be life-changing.

Lucy is a wonderful gynaecological nurse who has worked in sexual health, on a gynae ward and in school nursing. In her own words, she says she has seen 'thousands of vaginas'. She told me that there are many possible causes of pain during sex:

'It could be so many things, so as specialists it's our job to try and eliminate possible causes. It could be down to allergies, you could be allergic to your partner's semen, you might just have a small vagina and a larger partner and this is causing tears. It could be endometriosis, vaginismus, vulvodynia, pelvic inflammatory disease, an STI. It could also be gynaecological cancers, so it is very important to get any pain or discomfort checked.'

Her advice is to be as specific as possible when describing the pain to a doctor, as this will make it easier to refer you. Being able to answer questions such as, where is the pain located? Is there bleeding? Is the pain before or after your period? Does it feel like a cut, an ache or a burning sensation? From those questions, they will refer you to sexual health or gynaecology outpatients to have further tests.

If there is nothing physically wrong with you then potential emotional and mental blocks will be looked at. There is available counselling (although Lucy admits that it can be very difficult to get on the NHS). She also suggests online forums, which offer support, and information such as different sexual positions that can minimise pain and relaxation exercises to help with tension or anxiety around penetration.

Online forums definitely can be an excellent place to find support. I very much wish there had been more available when I was a teenager. I spoke to Lisa who runs the incredibly supportive community The Vag Network, an online space for people who are affected by Vaginismus.

Vaginismus is a psychosomatic condition whereby a person's vaginal muscles will involuntarily clamp up at any attempt at penetration (including cervical smear tests or the ability to wear a tampon). Lisa told me that vaginismus affects people in different ways.

'For some, penetration is difficult, for others it can be extremely painful and even impossible. There are two types of vaginismus: primary and secondary. Primary vaginismus is when the individual has always found vaginal penetration difficult or impossible. This is often discovered during an individual's teens or twenties when they first try to insert a tampon or have penetrative sex. Secondary vaginismus can occur at any stage of life, even after the individual has experienced a healthy, positive sex life and can be due to a whole range of things such as a traumatic event, difficult childbirth or treatment for gynaecological cancer.'

She talked me through some of the most common treatment options, which include psychosexual therapy and using vaginal dilators (a set of silicone trainers that gradually increase in size to get the vagina used to penetration).

'Psychosexual therapy is a common option which you can get on the NHS, however you can be put on a long waiting list. Going private is obviously the expensive option. Don't be afraid to ask if the therapist will consider a sliding fee scale – essentially to consider adjusted rates according to one's income or online therapy, which is cheaper than in-person therapy. It is largely a talking therapy and you will be listened to in a safe confidential space and given exercises to do to suit exactly what you need, interrogating any anxieties, beliefs and emotional factors that may be getting in the way of fully enjoying sex. Do a quick search on the CORST website, as it is important to get someone accredited and qualified.'

'Dilating might seem daunting at first,' she continued. 'For someone who couldn't insert my little finger into my vagina without it clamping up, I am now able to use the largest dilator and enjoy the experience at the same time. My advice would be to set your own goals, be patient with yourself and incorporate pleasure into the experience otherwise it will feel clinical and too much like homework.'

I think it is very probable that as a teenager I had primary vaginismus and having someone such as The Vag Network to talk to about my experiences, rather than a doctor telling me, 'You just have a very underused vagina, it's very springy, get out there and use it more', might have meant years of not feeling so alone.

Anyway.

There I was in my friend's pristine flat, venting about the doctor I'd just seen, furious at him asking about whether or not I'd heard of masturbation and knowing that I was going to need more than 'good luck' to get me through. I stopped for breath and took a sip of air from my now empty wine glass.

I was grateful for the chat, aware that maybe I've said too much and perhaps I ought to change the subject to something less about my vagina, just for a little bit.

ME: Thanks for listening, I just needed to get it off my chest.

HIM: Wait Fran, hold on one second. That is sad Fran, that is really really sad.

ME: No, it's not sad, it's—

HIM: No, Fran, I am personally devastated. Ok so, who are you sleeping with?

ME: Well—

HIM: Amateurs, right? And look, I'm just saying this as a friend. And it wouldn't be weird. It wouldn't be, I

can 100% promise you that it would not be weird.
But there has never been a woman who I have not
personally satisfied.

ME: Oh, that's—

HIM: I love it Fran, I love vagina, in some ways Fran, I
am vagina. I am the Chris Martin of Vaginas, Fran; I
can *fix* you. It wouldn't take much, I think you'll find
I'm not like other lovers . . . I'm just saying maybe
you aren't broken, maybe you just haven't tried the
right penis yet . . . I mean you haven't tried *mine* . . .
yet. It's a magic penis.

He gestured to his crotch like someone on the shopping
channel displaying their wares. He gestured again, perhaps
just to check that I'd caught his drift. And a third time. I
had caught his drift. He stood up and walked to the doorway where he stopped and posed.

HIM: Do you want to come . . . upstairs?

He was leaning in the doorway, silhouetting himself, like
someone who has practised being sexy; he blew his fringe
up and looked directly into my eyes.

'I'm alright thanks,' I said, replying very quickly, 'but
thank you . . . thanks. That's a really lovely, *lovely*, nice,
kind, nice, *nice* offer. Thank you.' I stood up and immediately asked, 'Shall I put the kettle on?'

And I did. I went and put the kettle on. A close friend
offered me his penis and I made two cups of herbal tea, bag still
in. He came and sat back sheepishly on the sofa and we carried
on chatting as if nothing had happened, sipping scalding tea
and not mentioning my vagina again.

As soon as seemed polite I made my excuses and left.

I wish I could say he was the only friend to offer me their magic penis.

* * *

Erotic Fiction & Audio Erotica

My first memory of pornography is feeling incredibly threatened by it. I remember seeing my teenage boyfriend's browser history and feeling hugely wounded because the porn he was watching was nothing like me. (I am never, as hard as I try, going to be a triplet.) Once I knew what sort of porn he was watching, I felt an unattainably high standard had been set, I had to be as good as the porn, I had to give triple the energy. On top of that so much porn contains violence, humiliation and fetishisation of race, so porn has always been something I've always felt conflicted and confused about.

I'd click between videos with one eye covered, hoping to avoid anything upsetting and trying to make sure that everything looked consensual, already worrying about clearing my browser history from the first thrust. If you are wanting to watch porn, I'd strongly suggest paying for ethical porn, where consent, safety and welfare is prioritised. There's no shame in watching it; it's fun and can allow you to explore different sexual tastes. (Apologies to my teenage boyfriend, I now know that our porn preferences can be completely different to our dating desires, I didn't ever need to be a triplet.) If watching porn isn't for you, then I would highly recommend reading some erotic fiction or listening to audio erotica.

Reading Erotic Fiction

I'm a big reader, I love words and stories, so I don't know why I didn't think to read erotica until now. I definitely enjoy getting flustered when a chapter gets unexpectedly sexy and some of the books I read as a teen definitely fall incriminatingly open on the saucier pages. Even with those strong indications that this would be something I'd like; I'd never read erotic fiction for pleasure. I think my impression was that erotica would all be men in jodhpurs taking their lovers for a canter in the lower field or being made love to on a beach to the sound of soft waves by the new lifeguard with a mullet . . . I guess I thought it would all be cheesy and set in the past. And while there is a lot of 'giddy up' in saddle action out there, there is so much more. Reading erotica helped me connect with my own imagination and actually develop a sense of fantasy. If there was something I didn't like I could stop reading immediately and had more control over the situation. This did happen a few times, the use of certain vocabulary would turn me off, but this made me think about writing some of my own erotic fiction, where I can create a world that I'll really enjoy.

Audio Erotica

Unlike reading erotic fiction, audio erotica is hands-free, which is useful if you wish to touch yourself.

I opted for a story on the theme of submission, something that I think in visual porn I'd be wary of watching in case it was violent, but in audio version felt safe. The story left a lot of room for me to imagine my own surroundings and I even got onboard with the ASMR (Autonomous Sensory Meridian

Response) breathing and panting sounds (although I did get distracted thinking about the incredible quality of their micro-phones and recording equipment . . . what were they using to get such booming resonance?).

It was very immersive with the other character talking directly to me, so I was thrust very literally into the heart of the narrative. The only drawback was suddenly being confronted with language or words that I didn't find sexy . . . I didn't want my 'pussy' to be referred to as a 'tight little pussy', but it did help me think about what vocabulary I *do* like. This one was around eleven minutes long and, in all honesty, that's just not going to be enough time for me to even start to relax. So, as he (my audio lover . . . let's call him Ken) raced towards his climax I got a bit annoyed . . . he was going to come and then what? Leave me in an empty silence fumbling to rewind the track? I thought we were in this together for *my* orgasm, even though I had an actual body and he was just a disembodied voice. Story of my life. I now know I need more time to allow myself space to relax and engage with the story.

Listening to this certainly felt incredibly sensual and, with my headphones firmly plugged in, there were no worries about being overheard or someone seeing what I was watch-ing. Turns out privacy is a real turn-on.

HONEST CONVERSATIONS ABOUT SEX
Sex is unfortunately fortunate

A: Woman, she/her, straight, 29
B: Man, he/him, straight, 32

A: We got together when I was 19, I had never been on a proper date. My friend warned me he was a scallywag.

B: I didn't want you to think I was a scallywag . . . so we waited over a month to have sex. I was very keen that it wasn't going to be a one-night stand.

A: Sex was tricky.

B: When I was younger my foreskin came back during sex, and it was very painful, really tight. It had put me off sex, and I developed this mental block. There was always this voice in my head saying, 'Remember that time when this really hurt'.

A: I thought that it was that he didn't want to have sex with me, specifically me, but it was just sex in general he was worried about.

B: We had a bit of therapy.

A: Sex wasn't something I felt particularly comfortable talking about so I felt like we needed a therapist there to help us. It was really quite expensive for us; private therapy is not cheap . . . but it was good to talk.

B: I spoke to my doctor and went at it from a medical standpoint too. I thought if I get circumcised then that would help me deal with the problem head on. There were other options but this was the quickest option to getting me sorted.

A: There was a recovery period, then we thought 'let's crack on', but it then turned out sex was incredibly painful for me . . . can you guess where this is heading? It turns out that the situation had given me secondary vaginismus. I associated sex with being painful, so it had become painful for me. After the circumcision, in my mind we were going to go gallivanting off having sex everywhere, so it was a real shock when we attempted it and it didn't work.

B: We've really learnt to do things outside of the 'traditional' intercourse. But that saying, this summer we had our ten-year anniversary . . . we went away and ended up having penetrative sex for the first time.

A: In ten years.

B: In a long time. We had a big long bath, we'd had a few drinks in the bar.

A: We took all the pressure off, because a lot of the time if you are like, 'Ok, it's going to happen tonight' it doesn't happen.

B: We are now more interested in sex than we've ever been.

A: But it only really works because we've both had problems, we are unfortunately fortunate. I hated the dilators so much, stupid, plastic, not fun. I don't know why they don't just say go and buy a load of vibrators and just enjoy yourself. I bought vibrators the same size as my dilators, super skinny and thin.

B: If something goes wrong with penetrative sex, we'll just give pleasure in different ways.

A: I do want to be able to get pregnant, but I don't want to put pressure on sex having just started to enjoy it. I had to tell my mum and sister, 'By the way I've got a problem with my vagina at the moment, so getting pregnant might take longer than you think it should.'

B: I didn't speak to many people about it. I did want to have a conversation with somebody about it, but it's hard to admit what's going on.

A: I'd talk to my friends and they'd say, 'it's weird that you guys don't have sex' and I'd be like, 'we do have sex, we do, we absolutely do, it's just . . . different'.

B: It's our sex life, it's not the porn people see on laptops, it's not what our friends say or claim or pretend sex is, our sex is just for us.

6

Female Sexual Dysfunction & The Yoni Egg

'Yeah, I'm just not enjoying sex really, I guess I thought it would be this big fireworks event but actually I'm finding it really underwhelming and I end up pretending to enjoy it most of the time and it can be quite painful . . . sorry, how much is that? £4.99, great, and yes, I would love a *bag for life* please.'

Talking about my vagina had become oddly addictive. Even after my awkward friend in the doorway had tried to offer me his magic penis, I couldn't stop sharing. At work, BBQ's, on long walks, mid-meetings, at weddings when the happy couple are doing that long bit where they pose for photographs against gnarled-looking trees, I'd be nearby chatting about sex. If anyone sat next to me long enough on a bus or stood near me in a queue at the supermarket, chances were I'd start talking about it. This was for three reasons. Firstly, because I was finding it a relief to say it out loud: I'M NOT ENJOYING SEX. Letting it out into the world, not as this heavy secret I kept in a bedside draw next to unused bottles of lube felt . . . well, it felt liberating (or luberating, am I right? . . . maybe not).

Secondly, because people love talking about sex. They love hearing about it. Love sharing the tiny minutiae of it (all the while looking over their shoulder to check other people aren't listening to them talk about sex . . . but of course they *are* listening . . . because *everyone* loves hearing people talk about sex). It felt like many people had wanted to talk about it for ages and were really relieved that someone had finally brought it up.

Thirdly, it was incredibly addictive because for every person I spoke to I learnt something new, something which showed me behind bedroom doors and *do not disturb* signs that not everything was as perfect as I thought. I learnt about couples trying for babies where the sex had become a mechanical, scheduled, regimented affair, where the very thought of intimacy left them cold. I heard stories of dry spells, overly wet spells and spells . . . people doing actual magic spells on their genitals; chanting and steaming them with herbs to rejuvenate and reinvigorate. I heard a lot of penis worries, foreskin troubles, erection quandaries and, among all these stories, I was beginning to feel a bit less broken. Suddenly I belonged to this web of people who, ranging from sometimes to every single time, found sex tricky. It was a strange club to belong to but I was in very good company.

Admittedly among all of this, I received a lot of unsolicited advice . . .

ADVICE GIVER: Can't you just enjoy the sex you are
    having? I feel satisfied knowing my partner is satisfied.
ADVICE GIVER: Have you thought about becoming a
    lesbian? I hear there's less penetration.
ADVICE GIVER: Isn't it a bit hedonistic to be seeking
    pleasure all the time Fran? I find a lot of enjoyment
    from the natural world . . . do you . . . *ramble?*

Sadly, I still do not ramble . . . unless ramble is a euphemism for something else? In which case, the answer is still . . . *probably* not?

Despite these comments I was finding a sense of freedom in losing the secrecy and shame surrounding my experiences and realised that if I could be as honest with sexual partners as I was being with friends (and a nice lady I met on a night bus), I would be in a much better position to have sex I might enjoy.

I'd also started doing research, contacting specialists who might be able to point me in the direction of useful books, tips, hints and studies. I felt like a sex investigator pinging off email after email.

Dear Dr Genitals Expert, I read your incredible paper and was wondering if . . .

Hello Vulval Pain Researcher, your article really struck a chord with me and I was wondering if . . .

Hi Shamanic Vagina Whisperer, your website is incredibly well designed (I particularly enjoy the sound effects, it is rare that a website takes you so fully into the womb) and I was wondering if . . .

The more I was reaching out and starting conversations the more confident and hopeful I was feeling about sex. In this new positive mindset, I felt ready to give intercourse another go and this time be completely honest about my difficulties with sex, my future sexual partner was going to hear everything.

He was a friend, of a friend, who was incredibly comfortable talking about periods. It turns out there are few things

I find more sexually attractive in someone than a willing-ness and openness to talk about the menstrual cycle. We went on a long walk along the Thames and ate an ice cream on the river bank. He talked eagerly and empathetically about his friends who have terrible period pains, how he brings them hot-water bottles and painkillers and how everyone should have to stay for the period chat at school, 'Otherwise they'll never know what is happening in any of the bodies around them.' (I, by this point, was already mentally picking out the building we would wed in and on which day of my cycle I would wed him on . . . perhaps we would all just free bleed through the ceremony.) 'Yes' I thought, he seemed like a really good person to practice being completely honest with.

I decided if I said it all very fast then perhaps it wouldn't be so hard, and if I got it out between bites of ice cream, then we could always pretend I didn't say anything at all while chomp-ing on our Flakes.

'So, um actually, this might be a lot, a bit, actually yeah quite a lot of information, but, so, but, sex . . . uh yeah, the thing is that sex, it is hard, *hard* . . . no pun intended (because . . . erec-tions, they are also *hard*, y'know, sorry) . . . *hard* for me and sometimes, sometimes it hurts and I guess that means I find it hard to enjoy it and achieve . . . not *achieve*, complete? . . . resolve? . . . conclude, bring about, um . . . *actualise* an . . . a climax, an orgasm, a coming and then I guess sometimes I pretend to have actualised a . . . well, you know, more than I maybe have actualised and I don't want to do *that* anymore, I want to actually actualise.'

I don't know why my mind had settled on 'actualise' as a synonym for orgasm but it had gripped it, hard.

He looked at me unblinkingly. I stumbled on, willing him to blink.

'There's this . . . I guess, condition, FSD. It's not a disease, you can't, um catch it, it's just if you have a problem with . . . sex, with all the normal bits of sex, it's new to me and I'm doing a lot of research and I'm not sure how I feel about it, but maybe, maybe it might be a useful label to know because it means it's a thing, it means it exists, but we, we don't have to use it, not that we are definitely going to have sex, because who knows what is going to happen in life? I certainly don't.'

We were leaning on a railing, not quite looking at each other in the eye, but I saw him turning what I'd said over in his mind, as I tried to look windswept and casual, not noticing the ice cream dribbling down my wrist and into my sleeve.

'Thank you for telling me that. That's really . . . *something*,' he said, and then, 'I get it. I find it really hard to stay hard.'

'What?'

'I find it hard to maintain erections? Partners often think I don't fancy them, but I really do, just my . . . penis and my brain don't always feel like they are communicating with each other. For a while I just stopped having sex all together because the more worried I got, the harder it was to get hard and the less I wanted to have sex because . . . well it was embarrassing, not very manly. Have you ever just stopped wanting to have sex?'

I stopped and thought about this. Yes, I definitely had and I told him.

'In 2012, London's Olympic year (probably just a coincidence but who knows), I completely stopped wanting to have sex. My brain and body both wouldn't even entertain the idea in case it might be painful.'

Leaning against the railing, watching the sunset over the river, my date took a deep breath. 'I completely understand. Look, not to put any pressure on the situation, but I find you incredibly sexy and I really want to have sex with you a lot.' He took a long slurp of ice cream, 'And maybe, because we've both had problems, maybe we'll be perfect for each other . . . sexually. Because we both get it. It might just take a little bit of patience and we can really take our time to see what works, I'm not in a rush.' The words 'not in a rush' reverberated around my brain, like the sexiest foreplay there ever was.

'I find your honesty . . . incredibly refreshing,' he continued, 'it makes me feel very close to you and like I *really* know you. This conversation doesn't usually happen, normally there is very little conversation before sex and it should happen more often. It should always happen ideally. I don't usually tell people about my problem until after the first time it goes wrong, but that feels like I'm being dishonest. I feel really honoured that you have chosen to share this with me. Just promise me you'll keep talking to me and telling me how it is for you, I'll always listen.'

Oh. Be. Still. My. Fluttering. Vagina.

These were the words I had wanted to hear. He got it. He understood. He could empathise. Could there be a better sexual partner than someone who has gone through something so intimately similar?

A seagull the size of a small bear landed next to us and made aggressive eye contact, prompting him to take my hand and ask, 'Would you like to come to mine next week? We don't have to *do* anything, as I said before . . . I'm really in no rush, but there are some things we could try. I know what you are going through and I want to help.'

We aren't in a rush. We aren't in a rush. We aren't in a rush.

The following Tuesday evening I arrived at his flat in a trendy part of east London. He had perhaps too many cacti and not enough places to sit, but he looked overjoyed with himself.

'I've done a lot of research,' he beamed. 'Trust me, I read lots of articles and I think together we can crack this.' Giddy with excitement, he listed facts and statistics as he undressed, reassuring me that my pleasure was 'paramount' to him. I asked to use lube and he reached for it and when I say reached for it, I mean his own lube stash; he had his own lube in its own drawer. He applied it confidently, not breaking the moment at all. He asked me about birth control; we had a brief but mature conversation about it, which again, who knew that was such a turn on for me? We were two very responsible adults having responsible conversations about sex and it was no big deal. The dialogue was fun, considered and careful, with buckets of consent and checking in with each other.

'Are you ok?'

'Yes, I'm definitely ok.'

'Is this ok?'

'Very ok, are you ok?'

'I am so ok.'

'Ok.'

Tick, tick, tick, boom.

Then we headed towards penetration. I told him when it was painful going in and he immediately asked if he should stop. I shook my head and with a tender negotiation, he inched himself in and finally, we were there. It didn't feel great, but he was inside me and that felt like something to celebrate. It was uncomfortable but manageable, surely with this level of open communication I was about to experience the kind of sex I had heard people raving about.

'Ok Fran, let's see if we can figure this FSD out.'

His face changed, a look of intense concentration replacing his flirtatious glances. Suddenly incredibly serious, almost as if we were entering an exam.

FSD
Level: Foundation tier
SEX
Component 69: ARE YOU SEXUALLY DYSFUNCTIONAL?
Time allowed: Far too little

Materials
For this paper you must have
-A vagina that you think isn't working properly
-Low levels of desire
-Pain during sex
-Difficulty orgasming, please leave the exam hall if you think you might need to orgasm
-A scientific calculator

Your half hour to make Fran have a good time starts now, please show your working out and put your hand up if you require additional paper.

PRACTICAL EXAM

You may begin . . .

It was silent.

I had promised not to make any noise unless I really felt something. I felt nothing. The only noise was the soft squish, squish, squish of buttocks on mattress.

Squish, squish, squish.

It seemed to be stopping him enjoying it too.

Squish, squish, squish.

We studied each other's faces intensely, wondering if this was ok.

Squish!

The silence was too much to bear.

'Why don't we try like this?' he said, flipping me over.

Squiiiish.

'Or perhaps this will work better?' he intertwined his legs with mine in a new configuration.

Squishsqishsquishsquishsquish.

'I think probably if I slow right down'

Squiiiiiiiiiiiiiiiiiiiiiiiish.

'What about this?'

SQUISH!

'Or this?'

. . . squish.

'How about this?'

'Put your leg here . . . lie back more . . . scrap that, turn around, lean back . . . touch yourself, touch me, touch one nipple, clench, release, clench, release, clench, breathe Fran, breathe, be the breath.'

He became more and more exasperated by the moment, every thrust full of 'put your left leg in, your left leg out, in out, in out, shake it all about' energy.

I was so close to cheating on the exam and just pretending I was enjoying it. It would have been the easiest most familiar thing in the world. He was giving it all so much thought, military levels of concentration on his face, mentally ticking manoeuvres off the list he thought *should* work and then after a few minutes of trying he'd go back to the drawing board. He was looking at my body like it was a sexy escape room, a tricky crossword puzzle or a well-lubricated Rubik's Cube.

EXAM BREAK FOR HYDRATION: PLEASE DRINK ONE GLASS OF WATER

I caught myself making an 'OH!' noise out of old habit and quieted myself immediately. I felt myself arch my back against him sexily to *show* him 'it's ok', but he gave me a stern questioning 'is this real?' look and I immediately slackened. I wondered if smiling was allowed? Just something, *anything* to lift the mood, to show each other that we wanted to be there and that we were having a good time, even if we weren't having a great time. His eyes searched my face desperately for any visible signs of enjoyment or discomfort and looked more and more disappointed by the second. Eventually, after what felt like hours but was more likely around fifty-five minutes, he said:

'Please may I come?'

and I said,

'Please . . . *Please*'.

And he does.

No marks awarded. Candidate Fran Bushe has been awarded a 'U'. Sexual partner awarded an 'A' for effort.

'Sorry,' he said, 'and sorry for saying sorry. I was just worrying the whole time that I was hurting you and it really broke my heart to think it might be. Did it hurt? Was it nice? Even a bit nice? Maybe we could reflect on the bits that did and didn't work . . . for next time, so I can rethink my strategy, this isn't the end of this, we are going to crack it, goodbye FSD.'

'There's no point,' I replied, 'I'm broken. Even once I can get it in . . . it still doesn't *feel* anything. I'm just never going to be able to do this.'

We sadly and grumpily cuddled, neither able to meet each other's eyes. I felt my old instincts to cheer him up with more sex, but quietened them.

He sighed, 'I'm sorry I got upset. I just really thought I could do this, I've been where you are.'

'No, I'm sorry. I'm sorry that I'm not easier.' I picked up his sad sentence and then didn't know quite where to put it. It was sex by numbers, without the noises or fun sense of curiosity. We had tried so hard that we had sexed all of the enjoyment out of it.

'It's ok,' he said, 'I'm not ready to give up. I'm not going to give up on you. It isn't over until you come.' Taking a long swig of water, he visibly shook off his negative thoughts and might as well have been donning gloves and goggles, ready to get back to the sex laboratory.

'It's ok,' I said, 'we can try again later.'

'It shouldn't be over. It isn't over, just because it's over for me, doesn't mean it's over for you, how is that fair? Everyone should come.' His 'never leave a good orgasm behind' attitude was heartwarming but the moment had definitely entirely passed.

'I'm really ok.'

'Just let me try, being open-minded is the first step, I've overcome my problems and you can overcome yours, I read that if you believe that I can make you come then you will, just believe.'

I let him have a go.

EXAM RETAKE

He ends up doing the gentlemanly thing, and falls asleep fingering me.

MARKS AWARDED: 0

With this sleeping man tucked up close next to me, about as close as it is possible to be with another person, I felt incredibly alone, exhausted and bored of feeling difficult and complicated and dysfunctional. To distract myself I checked my emails, taking my phone under the duvet so as not to wake him. Among the spam was a reply from one of the specialists I had reached out to.

> Dear Fran, Thank you for your email. I'm afraid I have quite strong opinions on FSD. Making women think there is something wrong with them is dangerous. Everyone is different. All sex drives are different. Female Sexual Dysfunction does not exist. I've attached some links below . . . but please don't feel like you are abnormal or broken . . . you are completely normal.

This was the last thing I expected. Having just discovered this 'diagnosis' of FSD that potentially legitimised some of my experiences, I was being told now that FSD didn't even exist.

I felt like I'd just been submitted to the practical exam by the sleeping man besides me, but now it was time for the theory.

Instructions for theory exam
-Use black ink or black ballpoint pen
-Answer all questions
-Do all rough work in this booklet. Cross through all work you do not want to be marked
-You must answer the questions in the space provided. Do not write outside the box or inside anyone else's box

SECTION A
You have been studying the history of Female Sexual Dysfunction. In order to establish whether or not you are in fact dysfunctional please answer the following multiple choice questions

1) In the early 90s, a drug being trialed for high blood pressure gave the unexpected side effect of causing erections. This drug was called Viagra and made $182.2 million of sales in the first two months alone.[22] Using your knowledge of the human race what do you think the pharmaceutical companies thought:

    A) We should do more research on this from a woman's sexual health perspective, let's see if we can help the many women who are experiencing distress in their sex lives.

    B) $182.2 million!!? If we can find an equivalent drug for women, we, the pharmaceutical companies will be rich. Rich. RICH! (Pharmacists dance to 90's tunes in a flurry of dollar bills.)

[1 mark]

2) To make a drug equivalent of Viagra for women, first there needed to be a clearly defined medical diagnosis, because in the 90s there just wasn't one. A series of meetings were held to try and define a female 'disorder'. They were drug-company sponsored, heavily attended by pharmaceutical representatives, with eighteen of the nineteen authors of this new disorder (the sexy FSD), having financial interests or other relationships with drug companies.[23] Using your own knowledge does it seem right that the people who sell pharmaceutical drugs had so much input in creating and defining this new condition?

    A) Hmm, seems a bit shady to me. Sounds a bit like creating a condition in order to make money from medicating it. (Just look at those pharmacists dancing in those Viagra dollar bills.)

    B) Need more information please.

[1 mark]

3) One of the milestones in the making of the new disorder was an article stating 43% of women have a form of sexual dysfunction, this is the figure that is widely quoted today. This figure comes from a study where about 1,500 women were asked to answer yes or no to whether they had experienced any of seven problems, for two months or more, during the previous year. These problems included a lack of desire for sex, anxiety about sexual performance, and difficulties with lubrication. If they answered yes to just one of the seven questions, they were included in a group characterised as having sexual dysfunction.[24] Could these 'problems' be categorised as just normal fluctuations in desire?

A) Yes – Two months of stress can severely affect desire levels.

B) Yes – Two months with a partner who isn't sexually compatible can severely affect desire levels.

C) Yes – Two months during a particularly difficult time e.g. divorce or fluctuations in hormone levels, pregnancy, being a new mum, menopause, depression . . . these can all cause normal fluctuations.

D) YES – A study that measured problems lasting for six months (rather than 2 months) saw the figure of sexually dysfunctional women drop to 15.6%.[25]

E) All of the above.

[1 mark]

END OF SECTION A. PLEASE TURN OVER FOR SECTION B – BUSINESS STUDIES SECTION

1) If you can convince women who have perfectly normal fluctuating levels of sexual function that they are unwell and need medication, you could potentially make a lot of money.

A) True

B) Yes

C) Yep

[1 mark]

2) The first treatment for FSD was approved in 2000: The EROS clitoral therapy device. This was designed to increase blood flow to the clitoris, using a small suction vacuum cup. It cost $359 and had been tested on a total of twenty-five women.[26] Assess the validity of the claim that this device seems very similar to suction and air-pulsing sex toys available from all sex toy shops, suggesting pharmaceutical companies are making

people believe they are ill, when really what is needed is education, empowerment and to engage with the clitoris?

Remember to show your working out.

[10 marks]

Ask for additional paper at this juncture if necessary

3) Meet Sally. Sally has a low desire level at the moment and it is causing her distress. She's heard of a drug called Flibanserin (approved by the FDA for the USA in 2015). Trials showed that it gave women taking the drug around 0.5 more satisfying sexual encounters a month, when taken every day. She's heard it was rejected twice by the FDA on account of it being no more effective than a placebo and for having too many side effects, like drowsiness and sedation.[27] It was especially risky when mixed with alcohol and around 10% of women taking Flibanserin dropped out of clinical trials due to adverse effects.[28] Should Sally take the drug?

A) Yes

B) No

C) Needs more evidence

[10 marks]

4) Wait Sally, there's more evidence! The third submission to the FDA for approval for Flibanserin came from a pharma-ceutical company called Sprout. They hired a PR firm who set up an organisation called Even the Score, which were talking about levelling the disparity of sexual solutions for men and women. Sounds good, right, Sally? They led a fierce campaign with patient-focused meetings for women who were affected by low desire to share their experiences, gathering vast female support. The campaign was so

powerful that *Time* magazine listed the drug as the number one inanimate object that drove the news in 2015![29] Using the powerful and accurate rhetoric of gender inequality as the forefront of their argument, Even the Score heavily pressured the FDA into finally approving Flibanserin. Two days after they did so, Sprout sold the drug to Valeant Pharmaceuticals for one billion dollars. The drug went on to have none of Viagra's success, with low sales and many doctors unwilling to prescribe the drug due to side effects.[30]

Draw a fully labelled diagram of whether or not Sally should take the drug?

[20 marks]

END OF SECTION B. TURN OVER FOR SECTION C – QUICK-FIRE QUESTIONS

1) Is not enjoying sex a condition?
   A) Yes
   B) No
   C) I've no idea, sex is a bit physical, a bit psychological, but then there's a heap of social, gender and societal factors all jumbled up in there as well.

[100 marks]

2) Who gets to decide what is a normal functioning level of sexual desire for you?
   A) You do.
   B) Yup, you.
   C) You heard me, it's you!

[500 marks]

3) Is a lot of the problem not your body at all but actually mostly the society it exists within?
   A) Yes! Take down the patriarchy, I'll fetch a pitchfork.
   B) Yes! Teach everyone more about the type of pleasure that works for them.
   C) Sometimes it can be your body, but the lack of research and training means getting appropriate treatment is extremely difficult.
   D) AHHHHHHHHHHHHHHHHHHHH.
   [1000 marks]

4) What is a normal level of sexually desire?
   A) It doesn't exist. One person's rampantly horny is another person's dry spell. One person might expect to have sex every day, whereas another person is happy with once a week, or once a month, or never. One person might class successful sex as having an orgasm, while another might class it through duration of session, achieving penetration or having an active sexual fantasy one rainy Sunday afternoon. Some people might not want to have sex at all. Enjoying sex means different things for different people at different times, which is why it is so tough to measure.
   B) 3.14 recurring.
   [1500 marks]

5. So, are you broken?

Finish the sentence you are writing. Pens down. Invigilators will be collecting your papers.

In bed that night I closed the email, overwhelmed with

information. Even if FSD wasn't a real thing I still felt broken and that there should be support available, but from who? It hadn't felt like it was a doctor's responsibility and my own attempts to work it out had left me feeling like more of a problem. Studies say that good sex can help you fight the flu, prevent heart attacks, aids sleep, makes you look younger, live longer, boosts creativity, helps with stress, depression and can reduce pain by 50%. Reading that list, I wanted in. I wanted enjoyable sex!

The man next to me stirred and began to wake. He reached over and stroked my thigh.

'I'd like to try again, I've got a few more ways I can do this for you,' he said.

'Sorry, I need to leave.'

'What?'

'Mm yeah, I need to go.'

'But I want to make you come and then I want to make you breakfast . . . I specifically want to make you pancakes.'

Now, I love pancakes a lot, but I knew I couldn't get sucked in by those delicious breakfast items.

As he put on his clothes dejectedly I realised that this was what had to happen. I'd been trying to fix sex by having sex with people. I was right that when I turned thirty and became single, I had a great opportunity to learn about sex, but I'd started in the wrong place. I needed to start closer to home. With just me and my body . . . and a small purchase from the internet.

Two days later, my egg arrived.

The internet is full of solutions promising you a better, longer, harder, wilder, more pleasurable sex life. Travelling home from east London that morning I googled solutions to ignite my loins, finding a 'sex liquid' made from the bodies of beetles (sometimes fatally poisonous), an injection of your own plasma into your vaginal wall and articles about an invention called the Orgasmatron (surgically implanted and wired to the spine). As terrifying as these sounded, I felt so broken that I'd thought, 'Maybe . . . maybe.'

Then I stumbled upon an article by Gwyneth Paltrow's company, Goop, titled, 'Better Sex: Jade Eggs for Your Yoni', talking about the healing benefits of jade yoni eggs.

Huge disclaimer: Goop has since been fined for its unscientifically backed claims that these eggs 'increase vaginal muscle tone, hormonal balance, and feminine energy in general' and anyone who bought one was entitled to a refund.[31] Gynaecologists have concerns, that they potentially cause toxic shock syndrome, bacterial vaginosis and damage to your pelvic floor muscles. I sure wish I had known any of this at the time.

To a very disheartened Fran, who had just read the word syringe and clitoris in the same sentence, these eggs seemed to me like a crystally light in the darkness.

I'm usually quite a sceptic, wary of crystals, healing vibes and anything that feels like it only works during the full moon, if you've studied with monks for nine years and stared into the eyes of an ovulating panda. I hadn't seen any of the gynaecologists' warnings, so feeling very desperate I couldn't see what I had to lose. Gwyneth's jade egg retailed for $66, mine was . . . less. I ordered it hastily from Amazon Prime and it arrived in vast amounts of packaging for a minuscule egg. With it were instructions that the egg was to be inserted in the vagina for up to twelve hours a day after charging it in the sun or moonlight for a bit.

I decided to leave mine in overnight in order to get used to the feel of it inside me and to lessen the anxiety that it could just fall out, roll down a trouser leg, with a large clunk noise in the middle of my working day. The instructions said to slot some dental floss through the hole in the pointier end of the egg, in order to have something to grab onto to remove it. All very sensible. All I had to do was lie back, sleep and let the egg do its healing work. The next morning when I reached down between my legs to pull on the floss to remove the egg, the floss had vanished, disappeared entirely. Not only had the means of retrieving the egg disappeared but the egg had journeyed, moving up my vagina to a place where my fingers could not reach. No matter how hard I tried to get purchase on the egg it just stubbornly rotated, slipping away from me, further and further up. Now, I knew that the vagina is a cul-de-sac, so it wasn't going to *go* anywhere, but also, I now had an egg stuck inside me. I googled 'what to do if your jade egg gets stuck?' and I was in excellent company. This has happened to many *many* people; we were all in this together.

'Don't panic' came the voice of a thousand blog posts and panicky questions on forums.
'The more you panic the more your vagina will hold and clench onto the egg.'

'Ok great, don't panic,' I thought, 'I won't panic, the last thing I want is any more clenching.'
'Your vagina will hold onto the egg for as long as it needs to, but rest assured it will start to make its own way out once it's healing work is complete . . . it will probably descend in eight to twelve days.'
Eight to twelve days?!?
I imagined myself going to A&E telling them gingerly, 'I have a crystal egg . . . although I doubt very much that it is

actually crystal, probably just a shiny stone in the shape of an egg, because it was quite cheap from the internet . . . stuck up my vagina,' and the doctors crowding around tutting, looking at the egg shape clearly visible on the X-ray before sending me to the definitely overcrowded wing for idiots who have got things stuck up their vaginas.

I went to work, all day worrying that the egg was up there, praying, 'Dear Egg, please don't fall out in the middle of my appraisal, but also please do come out.'

The moment I was home, I decided I had to birth the egg.

I'd watched *One Born Every Minute*; I'd seen David Attenborough watch birds breed on various marshes; I knew how this was done. Squatting in the downstairs bathroom, I began to pant, trying to isolate the muscles of my pelvic floor and umm 'bear down' (without even knowing exactly what 'bear down' even meant, really hoping I didn't release anything else). The whole labour took about twenty minutes, before I heard the reassuring clunk of egg on Lino.

Many people swear by yoni eggs and can be found quite happily charging their eggs in the light of the moon (while I charge my laptop right next to them). So as usual, it's just really sensible to do a lot of research about anything you put in your vagina (or body), it's clear my pelvic floor did not agree with it and lots of experts don't either. The egg now sits as an odd vaginal ornament on my windowsill. (Yes, Mum, that's what that is.)

I had hoped that a yoni egg would start to build a stronger connection between me and my body, removing a sexual part-ner from the equation, but it turns out my internet crystal wasn't the right thing. I fell back into researching. I needed something drastic, something that would challenge my way of thinking and give me the tools to understand my body. After a few weeks searching and taking recommendations I found it and let my friend Laura know I'd be away for a week.

Morning Laura! Off to sex camp! Back in 4 days.
6.55 a.m.

* * *

Writing Erotic Fiction

After dipping into the world of reading and listening to erotica, I had a go at writing my own sexy story. So much of arousal happens in the brain, so this was the perfect way to tune into and curate something exactly to my tastes.

When faced with the blank page I felt overwhelmed and a little shy about where to start and so asked erotic fiction writer Tabitha Rayne for advice on how to begin.

Tabitha explained that 'writing erotica for yourself, simply to use as a way to connect to your sensuality or libido is quite different to writing for an audience. It can be very liberating and exciting.' I couldn't wait to have a go, so she gave me the following tips:

1. Give yourself permission! One of the biggest things that came up for me when I started writing was, am I allowed to write that? Well, I'm here to tell you YES you are allowed to write that! Let go of the thought that someone else might be judging you or the words that come out.
2. Don't try to write things that make sense or have good

grammar. If I look up from my fingers to see a jumble of red spellcheck lines and sheer nonsense, I get excited because I know, somewhere in there is something I lost myself in. I know it's going to be good.

3. 'But what I'm writing isn't sexy.' It doesn't matter, does it make you feel sexy to write it? What if it's the image of a paintbrush sweeping up a wooden gate or the smell of cut grass that makes your jaw tingle and causes you to trail your fingertips down the side of your neck.

4. Have a laugh! Honestly, if you're afraid that erotica is something serious, get rid of that thought. We've all had experiences that make us giggle or even squirm, it's all part of the fun. Some of my favourite erotica has that awkward edge, like bumping teeth when you kiss someone. Conversely, go deep and dark if that's where it takes you. You can explore your deepest places or just go on a crazy mad fantasy adventure with yourself.

5. Use your senses. Get deep into how every single thing makes you feel. What do you see, taste, hear, feel, smell?

Writing erotica is one of the most freeing, exciting things you can do by yourself and I can't recommend it enough for connecting your mind, body and soul. Here are some prompts to get you started:

That time I forgot to wear knickers . . .
I wish to be picked up like a rag doll and sail out to sea.
Bare toes on sandy beaches . . .

~~My Thoughts~~ My Inner Critic

Initially, I found it hard to turn off my inner critic, 'Isn't that a bit vanilla Fran? You could let your fictional lover do anything, ANYTHING and that's as far as you're going? That position is never going to be comfortable Fran, be realistic! How are they going to do that with all those tree roots in the way . . . what if there are bees?!' I kept feeling boring and unadventurous but I had to keep telling myself, 'If this is what floats your boat then that's fine Fran . . . it's *only* for you!'

There was also a lot of vocal consent in my story, a lot of suspense (it was a whole page before more than just the smallest bit of two ankles kissed) and a lot more fumbling with the clasp of my bra than perhaps necessary, but these are the things that make sex sexy for me. I like the personal touches, the bumping heads, the getting stuck in your clothes and the laughing, so much laughing. More than anything the story felt like me, my interests, my wants, my pace and my body. Here is an unedited excerpt of mine (the full thing is much longer) and I honestly cannot recommend writing your own erotica enough.

Nothing but the sound of the river and birds and breathing. And if anticipation made a sound then the air would be ringing with it. The space between their thighs more tangible than actual flesh. The place where ankles kissed a flaming beacon of, 'YES . . . maybe this is going to happen, maybe'. He looked up at her, his own face suddenly nervous. Was he thinking it too? Unsure if this was for real. His ankle shifted lightly, gently moving his skin gently up and down her calf muscle. Maybe just him being uncomfortable and bringing blood back to a dead leg but maybe . . . just maybe . . . he wanted to touch her. Just one finger on her skin and slowly with both her eyes trained on it, it smoothed a path up her shin. Sudden wind (oh my) made a shiver run down her back and still the finger rose over the knee and up, stopping just before her skirt. He stopped, doubting himself, eyes meeting hers, 'Is this ok?' he asks. She put her hand on his finger and gently guides it up and under her skirt. His fingers behind her, grappling with the clasp of her bra, fumbling, breath hot on ears, a bra suddenly thrown too close to the river . . .

That was my attempt at erotic fiction, try one of your own if you fancy.

HONEST CONVERSATIONS ABOUT SEX
Sex is messy and silly and exciting and fun

Non-binary, transgender, bisexual, 37

Speaking as someone who is trans, it's hard to find places where conversations about sex aren't problematic. But why shouldn't trans people also be able to talk about their genitalia and not feel guilty and talk about how sex feels and not be fetishised? People hear that I'm non-binary, that's my identity and they go . . . 'Yeah but what do you *have?*' If you like me, then what does it matter what I've got there?

I look a bit different down there because I'm on hormones and there's a bit of growth. Having testosterone makes me very sensitive down there and means I'm thinking about sex a lot. With transition my sexuality is very much in flux at the moment, I don't know which end is up.

I used to go 'In order for a healthy relationship I must be having regular sex constantly,' and this is what I've been told by the media. I'd freak out if I wasn't having sex two to three times a week. Sex is important to me now because I have a heightened libido but the shape of sex has changed, it doesn't have to be physical, it can be fantasy or cybersex or phone sex, as long as it's fun and there's laughing.

I take antidepressants, that can kill any libido you have or, in my case, I kept my libido but I couldn't climax and so for a long time I just gave up my orgasms. I still enjoyed the sexual aspect, but I didn't come. I had to explain that to people, because people will try really hard to make you come and you're lying there thinking, 'I'm done, there's something good on the telly.' And now because testosterone has heightened my physical sensation a bit more, I'm orgasming a lot more than I was before and so I'm masturbating a lot more. I'd given up on it but now it's on a semi-daily basis.

Coming out as non-binary and starting to take hormones I unleashed the bisexual side of myself; if homosexuality isn't accepted, bisexuality just isn't seen. I've let go of a lot of norms and made my sexual encounters mine, not dictated by anyone else.

Communication means open listening as well as open speaking, which people often forget. In the past I have been very open with partners saying, 'I'm transitioning and while I can orgasm now it's still intermittent,' but often people don't hear, 'if I don't orgasm, don't take it personally', so listen to your partner, to their needs *and* their limitations.

I get a lot of men who are trying to explore their own sexuality in one person by going, 'oh you're non-binary, I get to see if I'm bisexual'. My gender isn't up for debate, I'm a human, not genitalia, for them to play with.

My best sex advice is laugh, don't take it too seriously, people have odd bodies and silly things that happen and you're going to fall over, you are not James Bond. It's messy and silly and exciting and fun.

7

This One Time at Sex Camp &
Being in The Majority

Morning Laura! Off to sex camp! Back in 4 days.
6.55 a.m.

SEX CAMP???
7.00 a.m.

*YOU CAN'T JUST TEXT ME SAYING OFF TO
SEX CAMP!*
7.05 a.m.

Sorry Laura, do you want to come?
7.06 a.m.

Where is Sex Camp?
7.06 a.m.

Dorset
Just off the M3
Turn right at the Little Chef
7.09 a.m.

Hang on, can we circle back around to WHAT exactly is Sex Camp?
7.11 a.m.

*Here's a link to the **website***
7.12 a.m.

Is that woman painting with her menstrual blood?
7.17 a.m.

I don't know. Maybe. Probably, yes.
7.17 a.m.

Is it a cult?
7.18 a.m.

Fran, is it a cult?
7.20 a.m.

I actually had googled if it was a cult and the answer came back as a resounding . . .

Probably not?
7.20 a.m.

Text me when you get there and before you go to bed and tomorrow. I want to know everything.
7.22 a.m.

DON'T LET THEM FINGER YOU FRAN!!!
8.00 a.m.

Don't worry, of course I won't get fingered. Easy.
8.30 a.m.

So, I was sat cradling my overflowing backpack on a train to Sex Camp. This was by far the scariest thing I'd maybe ever done and I was incredibly excited.

I looked around trying to work out if anyone else in my carriage was going too, but I wasn't entirely sure how I would identify someone on their way to Sex Camp. No one was *actively* having sex in this early morning commuter train; there was no one even with a particularly lusty look in their eye. I wondered if perhaps as we approached our destination, people would stand up, hide behind their copies of the *Financial Times*, slip out of their grey suit jackets and navy pencil skirts from Next into flowing robes (highly accessible for sex) or pull down wheelie suitcases full of kinky paraphernalia from the overhead luggage rack as they left. Perhaps not.

I checked repeatedly in my bag that I had, in fact, brought pyjamas. (Imagine getting to a sex camp and realising you'd forgotten your pyjamas.) They were there, neatly folded; they were sensible, they were flannelette. My main concern as per usual was what if I hadn't done the right thing with my pubes (I was guessing it was a fairly liberal pube zone and so actually for the first time in my life mine were maybe too short if anything and I was wondering what I could do to make them *seem* longer . . . maybe arrange them? Backcomb them? Maybe mascara?). What if there was someone there that I knew? A friend? An ex? A colleague from work who I would have to avoid all eye contact with throughout all future team meetings, both knowing we had seen each other's . . . *bits*. If *bits* came out that is? I was guessing at some point during a week at Sex

Camp, *bits* would be involved. To combat my worry about *bits* I'd packed my dungarees, because as an item of clothing they actually made me feel very safe and in control of my body. I guess they make it quite hard to know where exactly my vagina is (you all think you know where it is, but the dungarees add an element of mystery).

I obsessed about what I would say to the taxi driver when I arrived at the station. It wasn't like I had to say, 'Take me to Sex Camp', the place had a name . . . but what if the taxi driver recognised the place I was going to and made sexy chit-chat when all I wanted to be was anonymous? Then of course I started worrying that everyone in the whole carriage knew where I was going and maybe it's me who had a lusty look in their eye.

An older couple sat down opposite me on the train and one began to proudly show me pictures of their grandchildren. I was bracing myself for the moment when they asked where I was going, but they expertly saved that for when both the ticket inspector and someone pushing a trolley full of flapjacks were at our table, 'Where are you off to? Somewhere nice?'

I'd had enough time between making adoring noises about their grandson's bowl cut to have formulated a very perfect sentence:

'I'm just off to get out of the city for a few days, clear my head, isn't it nice to get out of London, London can be such a lot, so I'm doing nothing at all really, relaxing, staying for a few days with a nice friend.'

I, of course, neglected to mention that the *friend* was 150 strangers (fingers crossed for strangers and not any of the teaching staff from the school I was working at) and their *house* was a Conscious Sexuality Festival in the middle of the countryside and the doing *nothing* at all was a week of workshops designed to reconnect me to my body and sexual . . . juices . . . (I mean really, I had no idea what to expect but the website did mention the word juices several times). I decided they didn't need to know these things and turned the conversation back to their grandchild's braces; won't he have lovely teeth.

I didn't share with them that in some ways this trip felt like my last chance to fix sex. This place had to hold the key, because well, if I couldn't fix sex at Sex Camp, where could I fix sex? After placing my yoni egg on my windowsill, I'd fallen back into an internet rabbit hole. I needed something without the pressures of dating or feelings or egos to bruise (including mine). I needed outside help; I needed a professional. Sex Camp. A week to concentrate only on my body and a place where I could ask questions and get answers directly from the mouths of sexual gurus. Plus, three meals a day, a wood-burning sauna and no Wi-Fi. What a dream! The price seemed suspiciously affordable, so thoughts that they might harvest my organs were never far from my mind.

Arriving in the small town's station felt too normal. No one got off at the same stop as me, so I was worrying that there was in fact no sex camp, that this was all a big prank or that I'd been lured into a trap (I had watched too many horror films where this happened). I eyed up the taxis parked neatly outside the station, but the anxiety of cab-based conversation actually proved too much for me and I set out for the camp on foot. That way I could take my time, assess how I felt and maybe pop into a corner shop to fill my backpack with few (many) cans of G&T on the way (Sex Camp was a booze- and drug-free zone, but I could always distill them into artisanal looking glass bottles and say it was an elixir).

'Are you going to Sex Camp?'

A very normal looking silver car pulled up beside me and in it the most normal-looking woman, with a very normal expression on her face.

'Fancy a lift?'

I decided she would be my litmus test. If in talking to her I realised that this place didn't sound right for me and she made any attempt to harvest my organs, then I could hide behind a tree when we arrived at camp and then turn immediately back around, back to the station, definitely popping into the corner shop for a G&T, despite it only being 10 a.m.

The back of her car was stuffed full with an enormous and highly elaborate bell tent, as she was a regular on the sex camp circuit. 'I do all of them,' she said. 'In the summer I just drift from festival to festival.'

'And in the winter?'

'Too cold for a sex festival.'

I didn't know if she meant too cold to go to festivals in general or too cold to take clothes off for sex, but I was excited to hear about the large networks of festivals. I thought it was a one-stop shop for fixing sex. Perhaps if this one worked for me, I would be spending my summers roaming like this, erecting buxom bell tents and doing up the inside of a cheeky VW campervan.

The woman was in her early forties and very laid back, the type of person that made you realise you've been holding a lot of tension in your shoulders and back and, well, everywhere really. She sighed empathetically at regular intervals, imbuing every sentence I said with emotional importance. A cluster of crystals hung from her rear-view mirror. Some of them looked suspiciously like yoni eggs.

'There's not many chances in life to truly explore your sexual and sensual body. I work in a very . . . high-pressured job, so

it's good to have these places to let yourself go, uninhibited . . .
you know?'

I did not know.

Her top tips for Sex Camp were:

- Make sure you are standing near someone you fancy
  before a workshop leader asks you to get into pairs,
  really feel their energy and check that you will gel.
- Bring your own sheets because they can't change the
  bedding fast enough for the rate of ejaculation, for all
  genders. (There was a laundry on-site if absolutely
  necessary.)
- Make sure you go to the Love Lounge. As much as
  possible. Go to the Love Lounge.

At this point, I had no idea what the Love Lounge was, but
my mind got stuck thinking about fluids on soft furnishings
and whether I had change for a washing machine in my purse.
But mostly I was excited, imagining how in just over a week
I could be a changed person, the sort of person who needs a
fully functioning launderette just to keep her well-used sheets
in check. As we drove through the gates, I knew I was taking
my sexual destiny in my hands, arms wide open, ready for
whatever Sex Camp was going to throw at me. And suddenly
it was so close and real and raw that I could actually hear it, I
heard the beating, throbbing sound of my sexual awakening . . . and it sounded just like, in fact it *was* exactly like 'I
Like to Move It' by Reel 2 Real. I didn't expect that to be
the sound of my vagina reviving, but then I realise that song
was blasting on full volume from the open windows of Sex
Camp. There really is no other way of telling you this, but

that *really* was the first song playing on the speakers when I arrived.

At the end of the long drive, amid fields of tents (ranging from one man cocoons to enormous village-size tent networks, complete with porches and hammocks) were revealed the sexiest of all buildings, portable cabins, a few marquees gently flapping in the August breeze and a large stone house, just rundown enough around the edges not to feel intimidating or too much like a National Trust property. Inside were occasional paintings of couples in thoroughly over ambitious gymnastic sexual positions, one involving various sea monsters and a coy carp. Everything smelt of cedarwood. I hesitated to sit down on anything, because my mind was still thinking about what had happened on those surfaces and how many clammy butts had been there before mine. I imagined it was quite a lot of butts.

From the first moment through the door, people *were* moving it and liking it. They were dancing, hugging, embracing, kissing each other. I felt like a new partner being brought home for Christmas, hoping they would all like me and approve of me dating their first born. I needn't have worried because they welcomed me in with open flailing dancing arms.

'*Welcome, it's so good to know you, to really know you . . .*'

'*. . . you are so beautiful . . .*'

'*. . . may I hug you?*'

'*Would you like a massage? . . .*'

'*. . . can I stroke your forearms?*'

'*May I share this exquisite nectarine with you, it's so . . . juicy.*'

The word 'juicy' echoed around rooms, everyone there was in search of something exceptionally juicy.

Within moments of arriving someone had offered me a sexual healing session, another had invited me to her tent for a *yoni* (the

Sanskrit word for female genitalia) de-armouring ceremony and a couple gently posited that if I fancied a night of wild sensual abandon the door to their cabin (number five) would always be unlocked to me. When I told people I'd come to Sex Camp for the first time on my own, their faces lit up in wonder and confusion and I was repeatedly told how brave, bold and valiant I was being. I didn't feel brave, bold or valiant at all, I was just a sexually dysfunctional, single woman alone at Sex Camp.

I had expected more people a little bit more like me, on their own sexual quests, hoping to fix their own vaginas, but I was in the minority. One woman told me she could come from just thinking about coming, and offered to show me then and there, and there was already someone taking a breather in the long grasses outside because all the sexual energy was just a little bit too much for them.

My bed was in a female dormitory. Six single beds, which, by the time I arrived, were mostly adorned by lounging women neatening their tie-dye sheets and changing into silky billowing robes. One pruned a bonsai tree she'd brought with her. I plugged my phone into charge and made a big deal about placing my completely natural salt deodorant on my bedside table; it really was 100% organic.

My bed was next to a woman who introduced herself as a witch and pointed out from the window her polyamorous lovers who were lying on the grass outside. I wondered at first if this was to warn me off of them, a way of marking out her territory, labelling these people as out of bounds, but she, perhaps sensing my thoughts (she was a witch after all), said: 'We are together in so many ways, and what's wonderful about being here is opening ourselves up to others, we enjoy seeing each other have a wonderful time in the arms of new lovers.'

The sound of a gong ringing through the hallways summoned us down to the large marquee, where we all perched on small plump red cushions for orientation. The woman from my dormitory sat next to me. Her lovers came and formed a circle around her, all making small subtle physical contact with each other; a hand on the base of the spine, little fingers intertwined, an arm resting lightly against a shoulder. Newcomers to the camp were asked to stand up and be applauded (although the applause was having the group twinkle their fingers at us while making shush-ing noises . . . clapping never happened at Sex Camp, it was considered far too abrasive). There were not many newbies and I felt like a kid on their first day of joining a new school, thinking 'I hope I make a friend'.

The camp leaders took us through the rules. I liked the leaders to varying degrees. One with a voice that filled every nook of the tent particularly riled me. 'I would like you to exercise common sense. Don't be stupid. If you find yourself invited back to someone's tent, know that they probably have one thing on their mind, so don't get there and be all surprised, that will cause problems, just don't put yourself in that situation. Be smart.'

I looked around. No one was objecting to this. I wanted to say something, to question it, to point out that, 'It is absolutely fine to change your mind at any point, any point at all, even once you are in someone's tent, even midway through sex, any time, any time at all.' Normally I'm sure I would have. But no one else was objecting. No one was raising their hand. Surely I couldn't be the only one who thought this sounded wrong?

'Be mindful of him,' the dormitory witch whispered to me. 'The leaders shouldn't really be physical with the campers, but he will try, he treats this as if it's a festival for him, rather than somewhere he works.'

That unsettled me, what if something went wrong? Who was in charge then? How could things be safe if the people in charge were not being responsible? How could they look after us properly if they were sleeping with us?

I realised at this moment that we had to look after ourselves here, because in the pursuit of true pleasure no one was really in charge, because being in charge was, I imagine, not very juicy.

The teachers introduced themselves one by one, describing their skills and talents, all being met with applause-shushing. There was a spanking workshop, an introduction to kink, a guide to cervical orgasm, a session which involved linking your menstrual cycle to your Google calendar and something where you get set on fire. Orgasmically. These all sounded daunting but I was raring to go, happy to jump into the unknown delights, so it was with quite a swift disappointing fall to earth when I learnt that the first workshop of the day for everyone was going to be . . . hugging. Not hugging with fire. Not even hugging with your Google calendar. Just hugging.

'I'm great at hugging,' I told Dormitory Witch. 'Really good, I don't think I really need to learn how to hug, I mean how hard can it be? It's just hugging.'

It turns out I did not know the first thing about hugging.

'Align your genitals, but do not press your genitals. Take three deep breaths, you will know when to end.'

Fifteen minutes later, the hugging tutor who had a long swinging plait was walking among us barefoot, correcting our sloppy hugging postures, rearranging roving hands away from buttocks and sometimes rewarding and celebrating couples who got it right by exuberantly joining in the hug and loudly sighing.

I was not one of these couples. I did not get a celebratory sigh. I'd been hugging wrong for years.

'You've been used to fleeting, tapping, barely touching hugs,' the tutor frowned at me, swinging his plait, eyes full of pity. 'You've missed out on holding firmly, tightly, breathing into each other deeply, HUGS.' I clung onto my partner trying so hard to get this very simple thing right.

'How long should the hug be?' I asked the teacher, notebook out, like a good and attentive student.

'Put away your notebook, you won't need a notebook here.' He prised it out of my hands before replying, 'You will just know when the time is right to end the hug.'

I tried again, disengaging when the time felt perfect and then was shocked to find arms still tightly wound around me. I regrouped, breathed and tried again. The next time I hung on way too long, clearly missing the cue that the hug obviously was done as my partner tapped me on the back to encourage me to remove myself. I was overthinking this very simple gesture that I'd been doing all of my life, 'Where do my arms go? How much pressure is too much pressure? Do I close my eyes like I've lost myself in the hug or leave them wide open for full intense connection?'

Turns out I did not know when to end a hug: nobody wants to be the dick that ends the hug.

As the session drew to a close my poor hugging partner told me it was the best hug he'd had in years.

'YESSS!' I thought. 'I have won at hugging! First step, hugging, second step, sex. This is a good sign that I will soon master sex!'

We were divided into tribes, a group of five people randomly selected to be our check-in buddies for the week. It was meant to be a small haven for us to spend time in once every day and talk was to be uninterrupted, no advice given, just a place for us to speak about how we were feeling and for us to be heard.

I found myself biting my tongue, wanting to tell people, 'It's ok, you'll be ok', then nod assertively and say, 'oh that actually happened to my cousin, so you'll be fine', but I didn't. This time was for us to be heard but also to listen well and completely. If we had nothing we wanted to say we could ask for touch: hugging, stroking, massage, whatever we felt we needed that day. I looked around and saw groups all talking, sharing, listening but also having their heads stroked, feet massaged and limbs tickled.

In my tribe, there was a man called Marc. He was broad-shouldered, with arms that were made for hugs. On his body was a vast network of tattoos, curly calligraphy danced around his joints and inked naked bodies arched across his muscles. On his knee was a tattoo that looked very much like a shooting star hurtling out of a vagina. He'd been to Sex Camp for many years and so this wasn't his first rodeo by a long way. I was so surprised by people who keeping returning to Sex Camp, I had thought people would be in, get fixed and then go out into the outside world, their sexual toolkits swinging by their sides.

'Why do you need to keep coming back? Am I going to need to *keep* coming back? Do you not feel you've learnt it all? Do you have to keep relearning how to hug every time?' I tentatively asked.

He laughed so loudly that people in other tribes turned to watch and when he didn't stop laughing, they joined in. Soon the marquee was ringing with contagious laughter at my question.

'You don't *need* to keep coming back, but you might want to. You will probably want to. And this isn't like school . . . you will learn things, sure . . . but it's a safe place for experience, with people who will understand that sex is just . . . *more.*'

'But you know everything about sex now . . . right?'

'I don't know the first thing about sex.'

Right. Great.

He answered all of my Sex Camp questions clearly and kindly (and I really did have a lot of questions), everything he said sounded a bit like it had been borrowed from a high-quality stocking filler book of inspirational quotes. I was not going to accidentally fall in love with him, I had come to Sex Camp for me, myself and only me (and a little bit for Laura who was living vicariously through all of my experiences by text).

Have you had sex yet?
6.09 p.m.

Tell me as soon as you've had some sex?!
6.11 p.m.

Are there orgies? I've never had an orgy but I think I'd be really good at it! It's just organisation right?
6.15 p.m.

Send pics!!!
6.17 p.m.

The gong rang again, signaling the end of the orientation session and the start of free time. As people began to disperse, I began to worry. My tribe were all leaving and in a minute I'd be completely on my own at Sex Camp. This wasn't a summer camp where your every second was catered for. I didn't want to be clingy but the thought of being completely on my own here felt quite overwhelmingly lonely.

'Marc,' I said, feeling lost, 'what should I do now?' He engulfed me in a hug, squishing my face against a pierced nipple. While there I tried to discern what his upper arm tattoo said and was sure I saw the word 'yoni'.

'I'm going for a sleep and then a sauna. I'd recommend the sauna for you, just relax, take it easy. People sometimes jump in the deep end too fast and end up too exhausted, too early, there's no hurry here.'

We cast our eyes left and saw people running around the camping fields naked and whooping. One of them was the lady who had given me the lift in her car.

Marc smiled. 'They will not be in good shape for tomorrow and tomorrow is when the real fun begins.'

I'd been in saunas before; it didn't feel too wildly out of the ordinary. It felt like an achievable and easy first step and so off I went. Well, I went to the entrance of the sauna, I *lurked* at the entrance of the sauna, trying to work up the courage to go actually inside the sauna, so mostly I paced in the entranceway to the sauna. I lurked because the sauna was a naked space, my *bits* first foray into just being on display, the place where I'd learn if I'd made any pubic misdemeanours. I watched other people slink inside, totally naked, confidently strutting, showering and standing in power stances made even more powerful by their total not giving a fuck at their own nakedness. They stood sensually scrubbing themselves, moaning while standing under freezing cold water and making casual chit chat with me, while I tried to look them dead in the eye and nowhere else.

'Are you going in?' said a man, with an impressive beard and with his hands on his hips under the shower.

'I'm a bit nervous about being . . . naked, with other people.'

'Get it over with, no one is looking, they are just bodies after all, everyone is just thinking about their own.'

'Would you mind . . . turning around . . . and not looking?' I asked. He smiled at me and averted his gaze, putting his face directly into the freezing shower and howling.

I dropped my towel, took a run up and burst into the sauna, hoping if I moved at speed my edges would appear blurred and my entire body would remain a mystery. Once inside I sat on the wooden benches, trying to arrange myself so I seemed respectable, presentable and tucked away.

Within ten minutes, I was sweating buckets, stretching out full legs akimbo and covering my butt spots when I moved to pour more water on the stove and fetching the branches for massage. Seeing so many different bodies, with the strongest possible emphasis on *different* bodies, was wonderful. No one was looking at my boobs or judging my body because we were all just naked there together. It was so rare that I am naked with someone, anyone, without there being the imminent pressure of sex. Here, I could just enjoy the freedom of letting it all hang out, without wondering if my body was sex-body ready or whether I was incredibly fanciable at that present moment.

Marc came and sat in the sauna post his sleep. I stopped noticing that he was naked after a few minutes. I felt like a clammy goddess and the thought of putting clothes back on seemed like a terrible idea. Why were any of us wearing clothes at all ever? Clothes were a cloth prison for our beautiful bodies! Marc leant over just as he was leaving and stated very matter of factly, 'I feel a connection with you.' I stuttered out, 'Oh, oh, thank you, thank thanks,' and that was that, he stood up and left.

Was I meant to follow him? Was he asking me for something sexual? Where was the post-declaration of affection kissing? Did connection even mean he fancied me? Connection could mean anything really . . . maybe it just meant, 'What a nice chat, let's be friends, I'll add you on social media, do you have a LinkedIn?' Maybe he thought we knew each other in a past life? This was new.

'Have you been to the Love Lounge yet?' asked the naked (but of course I was not even registering that anymore) man with the impressive beard. Whispers of the Love Lounge were everywhere. There was an intense anticipatory excitement about it, people couldn't wait to get there, were itching to get there. 'See you in the Love Lounge, Love Lounge opens at 11 . . . will you be in the Love Lounge this evening . . . Oh, the Love Lounge was so wonderful last year, I hope it has the same vibe, mmm, juicy.'

'No,' I said, 'I haven't been. I keep hearing about it but I'm a bit nervous to go in on my own.' A wave of, 'Ahh no, you must go in, it's incredibly friendly in there, you'll soon make friends, it's a very open space, the best way to go in is alone' swept across the sauna and I thought, 'Ok, I've conquered nudity in the sauna, I'm clearly on a roll, maybe I am ready for this Love Lounge.'

Half an hour later, I loitered in my sensible flannelette pyjamas – why hadn't I thought to bring a slinky robe? – outside the Love Lounge. Wafts of incense, the occasional moan of pleasure and soothing low music emanated from a small fluttering flap in a medium-size tent. From the outside it looked like nothing much at all, a white-walled marquee in the middle of a field, but this was the sensual palace that everyone had been talking about. I tried to muster my courage and take a run up, but I couldn't. People strode in holding one, two or three partners' hands, I didn't know how to do this on my own. What if I went in and everyone turned to look at me? What if I had to sit at the side and just watch everyone else getting frisky? Would I feel like I could leave or would that seem rude, seeing as I'd just arrived?

I wasn't on my own in this though. A man in a sequined waistcoat was doing exactly the same thing a few metres away. 'Do you want to go in?' I asked, hoping that maybe him and I could at least enter together, maybe pretending that we were together (like the plot of a 'so bad it's good' romantic comedy) so I could do the scariest step with someone else by my side. He shook his head vehemently at me.

'I'd like to, but I was meant to be here with my girlfriend,' he told me shyly, 'but we broke up a few days ago, before we came here.'

'I'm sorry, that's really tough . . . I guess this place might be a nice distraction though, right? A get under someone to get over someone type place, right? In some ways a conscious sexuality festival is the perfect place for heartache, right?' I smiled at him hopefully and thought I meant what I said, a field full of friendly naked bodies didn't sound like the worst place to be getting over (or under) someone.

'We decided to both still attend the festival . . . so she's in there . . . just not with me . . . probably with someone else . . . we've both said it's ok to be with other people while we are here, but now I'm actually here it's all a bit . . . much . . . and I don't want to be with anyone else. She seems to have gotten over me much faster than I've gotten over her.'

I gave him a hug. A proper long one, I breathed into him and this time knew exactly when to end: it was just obvious. We walked away from the Love Lounge and drank fennel tea, me telling him about my broken vagina. I was learning that there were many types of connection at Sex Camp, but most could and should be accompanied with a herbal tea. I told my new friend that sex had always managed to break my relationships, whether I was honest or not, it had always made me feel alone.

My new friend sighed deeply and didn't say anything for a long while.

'The way you talk about sex . . . it's always about feeling *broken* or about *not working* or failing other people. I wonder what would happen if you changed your vocabulary, thought of yourself as normal and functioning . . . rather than as a problem . . . maybe just try saying it, "I'm not broken."'

'But I am.'

'Gift it to yourself as an affirmation, tell yourself that you are a sexual being and deserve good sex.'

'I don't really go in for affirmation things, bit sceptical really.'

'Just give it a go, what have you got to lose? "I am completely deserving of good sex . . . I am alive with physical possibility . . . I work completely as I'm meant to."'

I said goodnight to my new friend and walked across the fields back to my dormitory. The camp was alive with noise; someone banging a drum, singing, lots of people were chatting and moaning and massaging (who knew that massaging had such a specific sound).

Climbing up to my dormitory, sliding past one couple massaging each other in the kitchen, almost falling over three lovers all stroking each other's foreheads by the front door and then stepping over a couple noisily but slowly sucking each other's fingers, I made my way upstairs. I wanted to shout 'get a room' for a joke, but I didn't, because no one here really had rooms; only a few had access to their own private spaces, unless you had your own tent.

I arrived back to an empty dormitory and a buzzing phone.

How is it going Fran?
10.00 p.m.

FRAN ARE YOU ALIVE??
10.10 p.m.

FRAN text me to let me know you haven't joined a weird cult and now have a tattoo of a giant vulva on your back?
10.12 p.m.

Are you having sex, Fran?
10.13 p.m.

Oh, my goodness! You are definitely having sex!
10.14 p.m.

FRAN if you've had any drugs then make sure you drink some water . . . unless it's the drug that is bad with water, in which case just pop yourself in the recovery position and sleep.
10.15 p.m.

FRAAAAAAAAN!!!
10.18 p.m.

I'm alright! Don't worry! I'm alive
10.25 p.m.

PHEW! Have you had sex yet?
10.26 p.m.

Nope. I'm just taking a moment on my own in my dormitory,
it's a bit overwhelming.
10.30 p.m.

I bet! Is everyone just shagging the whole time?
10.31 p.m.

No, no shagging yet.
10.33 p.m.

None???
I had a google, there's a Wetherspoons fifteen minutes' walk from
you if it all gets too much. Or if you need me to come and get
you at any time, JUST CALL!
10.35 p.m.

I will. Going to get some sleep, make sure I'm fresh and ready
for tomorrow
10.36 p.m.

It had gone 3 a.m. before anyone in my dormitory returned. They arrived sighing, peeling off their clothes and sliding into bed.

'Where have you been?' I whispered to one of them.

'The Love Lounge,' they replied, 'you should go, it's so . . . juicy,' and pulled down their sleep mask, signalling the end of the conversation.

I lay awake after their luxurious sighs turned into snores, feeling like the teenager who hadn't gone to the party. Tomorrow I decided I would be braver, tomorrow I would grab sex by the love handles and get this broken vagina fixed. I went to sleep whispering affirmations to myself, 'I am sexual . . . I am capable of pleasure . . . my body knows exactly what it wants and what to do.'

The next morning, I was full of a can-do attitude. I attended early morning meditation and didn't tell myself off too much when my mind wandered. I ate the healthiest of breakfasts and followed people's instructions to 'pay the wasps no mind, for they are all part of nature', as dozens of the angry-looking insects swarmed over my grapefruit half. I gave myself the instruction that I was going to meditate every morning and eat only fruits from the trees, because it was what my glorious vessel of a body deserved. The grapefruit was not quite enough to fill me up, so I secretly ate a Twix on the way to the morn-ing meeting, where at 9 a.m. the dancing started in the marquee. There was no teacher for this, just a topless DJ in the corner and an open invitation to start your day with dance.

I threw myself in the deep end but knew my body rolling and shimmying moves were a bit more 'night club dance around your bag' than soulful sex camp movements. The man from outside the Love Lounge was there, watching a woman slow dance with a tall man in a kilt across the dance floor long-ingly. I gave him a wave and bounded over to dance with him.

The morning meeting was meant to start at ten past nine, but it was now twenty past nine, which was fine, I was sure there was a lot of sex admin that day that was holding every-thing up.

Soon it was twenty-five past nine, half past, quarter-to and still people were dancing wildly, we were so late at starting to fix sex and no one seemed to care! I was worrying something had gone wrong, surely this would push the whole day's activi-ties out of line? Sex wasn't going to fix itself! I thought I might not have enough energy to fix sex if dance went on too long, I'd already eaten my emergency Twix for the day.

'Aren't we meant to have started by now?' I asked my dance partner.

'Nothing starts on time here, there's no hurry, things will take as long as they take. Relax. Enjoy.'

Eventually we welcomed one of the leaders to the marquee with our finger-twizzling applause and they talked us through the workshops of the day. There was a choice of three at all times, some requiring a partner, some not. Some asked you to bring your own towel, some didn't. Lube was always provided, even when seemingly unnecessary.

At the end of the notices, while the camp erupted back into one more round of dancing, I asked the leader what the best workshop for a complete beginner would be and he suggested the consent workshop. It seemed better than jumping straight into the eight-handed massage session. My consent education at school had been largely surrounding not getting ourselves into dangerous situations. Boys were urged to make sure *she* wasn't too drunk or they could go to prison. Girls were told not to walk down dark alleyways and that it was really hard to prosecute if we got into trouble. Essentially it was a young person's guide to not getting yourself in a difficult situation where something bad could happen to you, 'Give a clear no girls, else how are the boys meant to know?' Every second sentence felt like it was, 'Just don't get too drunk, or you'll have regrets', accompanied by a shrug.

Consent education was incredible at Sex Camp. In this workshop we talked about how there are many types of touch, but sometimes we don't think enough about who the touch is for. Sometimes we touch someone because *we* want to feel good; sometimes it's because we want *them* to feel good. We talked a lot about giving touch to someone when we didn't really want to.

Previously all I had considered was whether or not my partner was enjoying being given touch and had never really thought about how I felt in giving it or considered what I was willing to give. I'd had a lot of sex, that really, I didn't want to be doing at all, or let sex happen to me because I thought it was what was expected. The workshop was a safe space to practice asking for what we wanted, practicing saying 'no' and becoming better acquainted with tuning in to when we wanted to give an enthusiastic 'yes'.

Partnered with a much older man wearing a psychedelic T-shirt, I embarked on a simple exercise where we set our boundaries and asked for different touches that we wanted. The aim was to really think about what touch we would like to receive, as well as give, plus to notice and listen to the feelings that arose within us; for example, not just jumping into something because we were asked.

My partner told me he would like to put his hands under my top and squeeze my breasts and for me to lie on top of him, giving over my full weight. I told him it's not what I wanted to do but I would like a simple hand massage, just on one hand, probably just on the palm. I didn't want a hand massage at all, but I also did not want to do what he had asked for at all, and felt myself looking for a compromise. He looked hurt by my rejection, and told me that his marriage had broken down, he hadn't experienced any intimacy from anybody in years and that it would mean the world to him if he could just touch me. I could feel a biting point in me, wanting to be kind to this person, not wanting him to feel sad or lonely or embarrassed – and yet I didn't want him to touch me. It was a familiar feeling, a hardening in my sternum and a gut twisting when I was about to do something I did not want to do or have something done to me that did not feel entirely right. I had felt it so often over the years but never really paid it any attention, because I was always worried what the consequences would be.

I offered a different compromise: he could stroke my arms, well, one arm, which he eagerly accepted, and began to do. A few minutes in one hand skirted under my top. I didn't want it there but I didn't know how to ask this man to remove his hand without making a fuss, or a scene, and disrupting the class. Everyone else in the room looked to be really enjoying the exercise, loving being touched, giggling with each other. I thought about the hands put on me on nights out, colleagues invading my personal space, a man at the end of a date smacking my arse, having sex with people because it seemed impolite not to, having sex because we were going out and that's what you do right, even if you don't want it? In the workshop room all I could feel was anger at myself, why couldn't I just enjoy it? Why was I being difficult? Why couldn't I just kick back, relax and be a good sport? And then I was crying. This was so much at the heart of everything that was wrong about sex for me. I didn't know how to say no at all. I was too worried about the repercussions of my 'no' to feel brave in saying it and so I simply endured. Allowed. Permitted. Because it didn't matter if I was upset as long as no one else was.

Why was I putting the happiness of this man I'd never even met before in front of my own? Why was I expending so much energy trying to please partners, but not paying any attention to what I wanted? We were told to hug and thank our partners and I felt my body tense up in his arms, unable to hold him back. I wiped my tears on his aggressively bright T-shirt without him seeing. I wanted to tell someone what had happened but I didn't want to be a troublemaker, especially not as a newbie in class. I knew I should let someone know that I wasn't feeling alright, but I worried about upsetting the man I was partnered with. I didn't want to ruin *his* festival.

Hanging around to speak to the workshop leader, I wasn't sure what it was exactly I wanted to say, but it came out, 'I really struggle to say no and I've really no idea the things I want to ask for. I worry I'll upset people with my no and that they'll take it personally.'

He tilted his head and smiled at me non-judgementally. 'I get it,' he said, 'but *no* is really powerful, if you give someone a clear no, then it means when you say yes, they can really trust it and what a gift an enthusiastic yes is.' I was about to leave when he said, 'Come back and do this workshop again. Not today and not tomorrow probably. Let yourself breathe a bit. But do come back; you never stop learning these things, that's why we run this class multiple times. It is the most important one.' I left the workshop determined to practice saying no, to listen to that twisting feeling in my sternum and make my yes's enthusiastic.

My next workshop was an Energetic Sex workshop. This time I made sure I was with someone I felt safe with and so stood near Marc. His hair was tied up revealing a tattoo of two (probably) snakes kissing on his neck. I may have slightly misunderstood the content of this workshop. I guess I thought energetic sex would be athletic, bouncy, sporty sex, where everyone worked up a sweat and people pulled muscles. What it actually meant was having sex using your energetic field, so I ended up shagging a man in the heart using my energetic phallus (which is located in the middle of my very unenergetic chest), which I put in his energetic vulva (located in his chest). We sat opposite each other, with a metre between us, rocking backwards and forwards in tandem, imagining that our energetic *bits* were making love. Whooops and sighs of pleasure erupted around the room, everyone it seemed was loving this. I felt nothing. Well, I felt pins and needles, (apparently that *was* a good sign), but I could get pins and needles on my own, at home, in my own time.

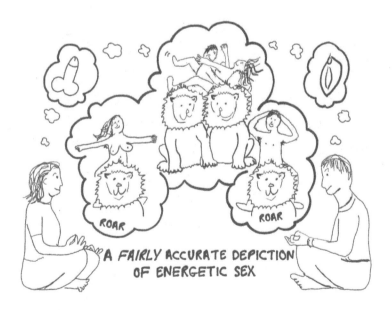

A *FAIRLY* ACCURATE DEPICTION OF ENERGETIC SEX

I was asked to visualise and describe my phallus: mine was thin, pale and flaccid.

One man put his hand up at the end. 'I don't feel anything, why can't I feel anything? Everyone else seems to be loving this, am I broken?'

This man was my hero. His voice meant I was not alone in not feeling like my pleasure invitation got lost in the post. I should in that moment have stuck my hand up too and shared that I also felt this, so that he would know he wasn't on his own, that he wasn't broken, we could have been a little team. But I didn't. In that moment I made a choice to sit in silence, part of the pack, not wanting to seem quite as lost as I felt.

'When do we get to the actual sex?' I asked the leader of the Energetic Sex workshop, who looked at me perplexed. 'We are already there,' she said and gestured her arm artistically around the room of energetic lovers.

'No . . . sorry, I mean *sex*, you know, the big S.E.X. pene-tration time, come on! (Yes, I sang this to the tune of 'Celebration' by Kool & the Gang.) It's called Sex Camp, so where is the sex?'

She looked at me kindly, 'Penetration is not encouraged at Sex Camp . . . If you really *need* to penetrate you can do that at The Cock Inn,' and cast her eyes out of the window across the fields, to an isolated caravan.

I walked down to The Cock Inn with Dormitory Witch after the class. It was the only place where penetration was allowed outside of people's own personal tents. Inside this cara-van were four thin mattresses on the ground, each with a thin opaque curtain between. It was cold, damp and felt like they really didn't want people to have penetrative sex here at all.

'Why the no-sex rule?' I asked her, sitting on one of the

mattresses and then deciding that actually the floor was probably a safer bet.

'There's lots of sex. Just less of the putting a penis in a vagina heterosexual kind of sex. It's about building up intimacy, and well penetration can be nice, but it's not all there is, it's a bit *lingam-*focused (Sanskrit word for penis) . . . most people with vulvas aren't going to climax from that anyway. I don't do penetration at all now, it just is a bit . . . inadequate. It doesn't do much for me.'

'Me neither,' I replied.

'You're in the majority. That's the same for most people with vulvas. You know that right?'

Yeah. Yeah of course I knew that. Yup. Definitely. Certainly. Yes.

I must have known that, right? At some point someone must have said that to me. Or I must have read it? Or heard it? It felt like pretty important information to know that actually I'm in the majority, that 75% of people with vulvas only orgasm with help from sex toys, hands or tongue. I couldn't have gotten to thirty years old without knowing this important fact; that penetrative sex just didn't make most people with vulvas climax. That was the kind of sex I was forcing myself to try and enjoy, time after time, and beating myself up if I wasn't loving it. I knew the clitoris was important, I knew it was something for people to focus on, but I didn't know that it was ok for penetrative sex not to be the gold standard, top shelf, Holy Grail sexual experience I was striving for. Why did no one tell me this? How did Dormitory Witch know and I didn't?

'Hang on,' I said, as she stood up and turned to leave The Cock Inn. 'Is there anything else I should know? I have a feeling there's a lot about sex I don't know and I had a whole week of lessons on the gall bladder at school but I didn't even know I had a clitoris until I was twenty-one and I'm still not completely sure how to use it.'

I waited tentatively, a bit embarrassed to have asked, but if you can't ask a Dormitory Witch at a Sex Camp in a caravan designed for penetrative sex about your genitals, where can you ask? She beamed at me and there on the floor of The Cock Inn, the Dormitory Witch gave me a better sex education lesson than anything I had ever had at school. It turned out she loved speaking about vaginas.

'Ok, so the clitoris is the main source of pleasure for most people with vaginas. It has absolutely no other function, nothing, zero, it is only for nice times. So trying to enjoy sex but not involving your clitoris is a bit like trying to row a canoe without any oars, against the tide, wearing oven gloves. I think you should probably have a really good look at your vulva, shall we get a mirror?'

'I'm alright thanks,' I said. 'I don't know if I want to *look* at it. We can talk about it without looking at it. I'm sure I can imagine it.'

'You don't like the idea of looking at it?'

I shook my head.

She placed one hand on her heart and sighed. 'I used to believe that my vulva wasn't attractive, but honestly the more you get used to looking at it, the less you will feel that. At some point I promise you, you will get to a point where actually you think it is pretty good-looking and choosing to know your vulva is beautiful in a society that will feed you endless messages about it being a mess or needing cleaning is actually very powerful.'

She opened her notebook and began to draw and label a clitoris.

'The bit you can see of your clitoris is called the glans, but the clitoris extends far beneath what you can see with your eyes, you can only see the tip, like an iceberg of the loins. Its full structure runs around 9cm in length and 6cm in width and looks like a wishbone. The G-spot is not a magic button in your vagina, but part of your clitoral structure.'

Her pen sped over the page, scribbling and doodling as her smile broadened.

'You can enjoy your clitoris through rubbing, tapping, making small circles around it, big circles around it, placing your palm on it and moving the whole area, pinching it gently, rubbing it against someone's hand, leg, tongue, mons pubis . . . sometimes it might be too sensitive to touch . . . sometimes it might need a bit of warming up, sometimes you might want to use something else on it like a sex toy, but until you know it exists you're going to be largely in the dark in enjoying pleasure. By focusing loads on penetrative sex, you are having sex that is the easiest way to make a partner with a penis come, but not you. One of the most important things you need to know is THE GAP.'

As we sat on the cold floor of the caravan Dormitory Witch explained to me the orgasm gap. Women and men orgasm pretty much at the same rate when they masturbate, 95% of people come in a few minutes from masturbation.[32] When it comes to penetrative sex in heterosexual relationships men still come 95% of the time, but women only 65% of the time.[33] But there is nothing wrong with these people, they can come mostly just fine on their own and women who have sex with women orgasm 85% of the time. Women come more often from masturbation, hands on their clit and oral sex than from penetrative vaginal sex.[34] If you add clitoral stimulation to penetration suddenly 73% of women are orgasming.[35]

'So, it's pretty clear that it's the type of sex that's being had that's making the difference,' she enthused.

'So, I should ask people to concentrate on my clitoris?'

She smiled at me gently. ' It doesn't have to be *just* the clitoris . . . you also have labia and a mons pubis and the crease between where your leg meets your pelvis is probably fun and nipples; your feet and toes can be hugely sensitive and, actually, your lower back and your ears shouldn't be overlooked.'

'My ears have always been weirdly sensitive. Are everyone's ears this sensitive?'

'Having your ears kissed might not look like what the textbooks say sex is but it doesn't mean it isn't sex. Don't compare your sex life to what anyone else's looks like because very few people are being honest about how sex is for them.'

'I'm in the majority?' I said.

'Yeah,' she stood up. 'You're completely normal.'

We walked away from The Cock Inn, me trying to look casual with my new 'I'm in the majority' swagger. I was completely normal.

'What would you like to do now?' she said. 'This time is completely yours; you can do whatever you want with it Fran.'

I thought about it. I'd drifted from workshop to workshop feeling timid and on the edges, watching everyone else enjoy their bodies. I'd felt lost and like I'd had my boundaries tested and disrespected, and now I knew that there would be no penetrative sex and that actually that was ok, there was one place that I really wanted to visit.

'The Love Lounge,' I said, confidently, 'I'd like to go to the Love Lounge.'

As simple as that, off we went, slipping our shoes off at the flap and sliding into the tent together. Inside was a sea of writhing bodies and soft moans. Massage bars were passed around freely; the lights were low and the pace was slow. There was a woman on my left having her toes sucked profusely and her boyfriend was on my right being tickled with a feather. With penetration of any sort banned in the Love Lounge, I was able to relax for the first time in a long time. I didn't have to worry about whether or not sex was going to hurt because it wasn't going to happen. I didn't have to worry about whether I'd end up in a relationship with any of them, because it was just about touch and being in the moment. Instead, I focused on being physical without any pressure of performance or expectation. Someone massaged my head, while another ran fingers down my back and the man from the sauna nibbled on my knees.

When the leader of the camp approached me and asked if he could massage my feet, I said 'No thanks, you're the teacher.'

'I'm not just your teacher, don't see me that way,' he replied. 'I want you to know I've noticed you and if you wanted to come to my room for some intimacy I—'

I turned my back on him. I did not want his intimacy and I was not worried about how he would feel about this. I folded myself back into the massage circle and warmed some oil between my hands.

That evening it was me sliding into bed at 3 a.m., sighing and glowing. I didn't look at my phone (which was also glowing) and fell asleep feeling a little flicker of . . . something.

The next day arrived and I was in. I had landed at Sex Camp. The oxytocin had hit. The cuddling and stroking had turned the entire camp into a sloppy slushy puddle of sex and happiness hormones. I loved EVERYONE. I glided instead of walked. I licked a man's face like I was a dog because that's what he wanted and I'd considered my boundaries and decided I'd like to do that. He tickled me for a solid ten minutes because it turned out that's what I wanted. I couldn't quite bring myself to call my vagina 'a yoni', but that was better than calling it a 'sacred space and source of life place'. Things were beginning to work and I was for the first time in a long time . . . wet. I sighed as I walked. I got a bit aroused singing a song about my dead ancestors to a tree.

Marc and I spent hours lying in fields, caressing each other's hands and only our hands, and looking at glow-worms down country lanes (not a euphemism, actual glow-worms). He told me that after many years of practice he could orgasm multiple times without ejaculating and I told him I loved him despite only knowing him for a few days. It felt a lot like love.

Fran! What have you been up to?
9.00 p.m.

Oh Laura! Wow. Honestly, I am so full of sexual energy! [emoji with insane heart eyes]
9.10 p.m.

Sexual energy?
9.12 p.m.

It's quite addictive, I'm full of oxytocin, I've fallen in love with a man called Marc, he is EVERYTHING.
9.13 p.m.

You've only been there four days!
9.13 p.m.

I'm a changed woman! Marc says that I am a goddess and that his body is only there to serve my body and that my vulva is a rosebud just opening. I don't know how I will be parted from him

when this is over, so I might have to move to Whitstable where he lives.
9.15 p.m.

Marc also practices non-ejaculatory sex, so he can come over and over again, so that his orgasm doesn't stop sex! He is amazing! He says he's going to get a tattoo of my essence on his inner thigh.
9.15 p.m.

I've learnt SO MUCH about connection and how to let go and slow down and intimacy, I've done so much crying, but I am working! MY BODY IS WORKING!
9.15 p.m.

Also, Laura did you know that I AM IN THE MAJORITY!
9.15 p.m.

Laura?
9.15 p.m.

Laura?!
9.16 p.m.

Are you sure this isn't a cult Fran?
9.20 p.m.

I was in love with Sex Camp. We talked about orgasms, bodies and our sexual anxieties over breakfast. We moved A LOT. There were naked saunas long into the night with no one caring about their sweaty bodies and wild, free pubic hair. I *was* worrying that I'd accidentally joined a cult but also knew that my body was beginning to feel *more*. I moved slower, ate slower and touched others slowly but often. I'd been fixating on penetration for so long, I'd made it my only goal, ignoring so many other types of touch, stimulation and experience. I began to understand I needed to slow right down to start to enjoy my body. Food tasted better, brighter, I watched the breakfast wasps dart around my food with a new appreciation and wonder. This could only be the beginning of exciting things . . .

THANK YOU FOR YOUR TIME AT SEX CAMP FRAN, PLEASE LEAVE THE CAMP NOW.

ME: Um, hi, sorry, I can't leave the camp yet, I've actually just started functioning. My body is feeling good, I'm in love with this man I met a few days ago and . . . gosh, sorry this is an overshare, but I'm really . . . wet . . . all the time.

PLEASE LEAVE THE CAMP NOW.

ME: Can I stay a few more days?

PLEASE LEAVE THE CAMP NOW.

I'd booked for four days. That time was now up. I wanted to stay longer, but I found out that all the dormitory beds were booked up for the next week. I prepared myself to bid farewell to the camp and the man I was certain after four days was absolutely my soulmate.

At this point I really should have just gone home. But I didn't. I strode down to the local village. I told myself that if the local village shop had a tent (highly unlikely as it was the sort of place that only sold fishing tackle and bubble gum) then I would stay, and if it didn't, I would go back to London and vow to try and hold onto my new slower, more spiritual, wetter self as hard as I could. The truth I wasn't admitting was that even though I knew that there was so much sensuality to be found outside of penetrative sex . . . I still wanted to have penetrative sex to see if I was truly fixed. I couldn't completely let go of the idea that it was 'the one true sex'. So, on the last day of camp, I walked down past the Wetherspoons and the café (where many of the Sex Campers had snuck for secret fry-ups . . . giving each other conspiratorial nods in there, sausages hanging from our mouths) and into the shop.

And there it was.

One tent left.

One tent in the entire village.

It was red.

* * *

Bossy Massage

This is a partner exercise, but it doesn't have to be a romantic or sexual partner, it can be someone that you trust and feel comfortable with. This is a massage that is entirely guided by you. Normally during a massage, we switch off, giving over authority and control largely to the masseuse, but not in a Bossy Massage. In this exercise, developed by American Sexologist Dr Betty Martin, your masseuse follows your exact instructions as to where and how you would like to be touched and this is the only touch you will receive.[36] The person giving the massage should also consider where and how they are comfortable touching you. It calls upon you to take charge of your experience and ask for only the touch that you actually want. It also means you have to be specific about details such as pressure, type of touch and duration. Examples of phrases that could be helpful during the massage are:

For the receiver:

'I would like you to gently tap my forehead.'

'I would like you to run your fingers down my forearm, with a medium pressure until I say stop.'

For the giver:

'I would like to touch you on the shoulders.'

'I want to tug gently at your hair.'

'I don't want to touch your arms, but I would like to stroke your feet,'

You can also practice adjusting your requests:

'Less pressure with your left hand.'

'Tap more quickly on my back.'

'Please put socks on me, my feet are cold.'

I have to admit the first time I did this exercise I panicked and completely froze. I was so unused to knowing and asking for what I wanted and so used to handing over all responsibility and autonomy to the person touching me. I found I was worried about them judging me for what I asked for. I didn't want to put them out so I didn't ask at all. While it was difficult for me, it was fantastic practice at saying and hearing no but also the thing we perhaps talk less about, being able to hear 'no' and it not be a big deal. We all know we should be able to do this, and not take it personally, but it is always worth practising in a non-sexual space like a Bossy Massage.

HONEST CONVERSATIONS ABOUT SEX
Sex is like chickpeas and wearing hats

A: Male, heterosexual, he/his, 45
B: Female, heterosexual, she/her, 44

A: We met at a festival. We were reborn in a teepee and did an all over body orgasm workshop, as you do.

B: He pitched a tent next to me. I wasn't very good at pitching tents, I didn't even have a mallet.

A: I'd bought a bell tent so I could cruise around festivals finding women ... and it obviously worked. You stole my welly and made me go into a naked sauna.

B: Six months later I got pregnant, so we went from cruising around trying to be in an open relationship, having lots of sex, to suddenly being a suburban family of four.

A: We play with different things that help us to get in the mood and connect.

B: We are quite good at orgasming. I think it's my superpower. I'm really good at orgasms.

A: We do the Wim Hof method of breathing and it just works for us.

B: Rather than say, 'Shall we go and have sex?' I'll be like, 'Shall we breathe later?' It resets us from that slobby parent, home-domestic-washing-up-putting-children-to-bed thing, to feeling much more in our bodies.

A: We feel the impact if we don't. Over the summer, sex dropped out and we felt we were holding our breath. The kids were going to bed too late. It's a small flat.

B: I think if we aren't having it every week it begins to affect us.

A: It's a bit like eating lentils or wearing hats, you forget to do it and when you do it, you're like, 'Oh, I should do this more often'.

B: You just said that sex is like wearing hats or eating lentils.

A: You know, when you wear a hat you think, 'I should wear more hats'. The secret to great sex is just getting yourself out of the way, let the ego go and be in the moment.

B: Sex is spiritual. I'd been raised a catholic so had thirteen years of nuns teaching you a vow of chastity ... and then I had these amazing, transformative experiences, sexually, and it felt the opposite of that, like it is actually bringing you closer to a sense of the divine.

A starts eating a banana

A: I always ask, 'How do we make this experience glorious?' We as people continuously stop ourselves having all-over, full-body orgasms because of the way we hold our body, but you have to move and make sound and it will happen.

B: I used to just tense everything up and stop breathing to orgasm and once I really breathed into it and kept breathing, I could flow my energy. I feel a bit funny in my body just even talking about it now.

A: You do need to make sound and movements to have orgasms, but I would never suggest anyone fake them.

B: It can start you off though. I make all sorts of noises, sex is one time you can get in touch with that animal part of you and not really care about being civilised.

A: We have to close the windows beforehand.

8

Meeting My Vagina & The Reverential Homecoming

CUE FANFARE: I was going to have sex. Penetrative sex. Going all the way. At Sex Camp. With Marc, the man I'd fallen head over heels in love with in under a week. In a tent.

Marc knew this was on the cards, because when I returned to camp, red tent under my arm, I had casually, smoothly and coolly mentioned it as we erected the tent together.

'Marc, umm you are a lovely fellow sex camper with whom I've developed a . . . *connection* . . . a big connection and seeing as I'm staying an extra week and I bought this lovely tent, I think it would be really nice, maybe, if we maybe . . . if we did a bit of . . . penetration . . . just a soupçon of penetration . . . I know, I KNOW, penetration isn't really encouraged here, very frowned upon, but I have a very small window in which to get this right. I could dry up again the second I leave camp . . . (Speaking of which, how long can I actually stay for? Another week? A month? Forever?) So, I guess I want to give it a go while my body is . . . *working* . . . and so what I'm trying to say is would you like to come back to my tent for some PENETRATION?'

'I'd love to,' Marc said.

He promptly disappeared and returned hand in hand with Dormitory Witch. For a moment I thought he'd brought her as an active participant in our forthcoming sex, but he promptly said:

'She's here to bless the tent, I don't want us to have sex somewhere that isn't special, and no offence, but your tent doesn't feel very . . . special.' I was delighted as they both set about making my £30 tent a special sacred space, smudging it with sage, chanting tiny chants around the tent pegs and wafting away any bad energy from my sleeping bag. Eventually Dormitory Witch left and it was just Marc, me and a very fresh feeling tent . . .

Guide to having sex, the Sex Camp way!

1. Look into your Beloved's eyes and get ready to put the nasty back in Namaste. Do not break eye contact, feel that sweet release of oxytocin as you stare deeply, cue feelings of trust/emotional closeness/wanting to be enveloped by the entirety of their soul.

2. Check that your chakras are balanced and aligned. Get ready to levitate as you bump and grind, but not for another 90 minutes. No rushing. Sit, breathe, sigh, but do not touch. If available bang a tiny gong or finger a wind chime.

3. Ok, it's time for some sex to commence, get ready to merge your spiritual vessels. Let your lover place any crystals of importance to them around the tent . . . if unsure of good crystals you can't go far wrong with a good classic bit of rose quartz.

4. At this point it is perhaps worth questioning if this is in fact a cult. But know that if it is a cult then I guess it's a cool cult?

5. Clear your mind of all distractions. You are Gods and Goddesses. Know that this sex is going to be the best sex ever, because you have done everything right. Stop thinking about how flammable the inner lining of the tent is next to those tealights and incense sticks. Maybe move any real fire hazards before penetration commences.

6. Safety first. Just because you are about to commence the most sacred union don't forget about contraception, although you may need to remind your lover to put that lingam in some spiritual robes (or an in-date condom). When your lover looks askance at you, like a condom may totally ruin your inner connection stay firm and remember:

    Ancient oak tree leaf = not a condom

    Goat skin = not a condom

    Rain = Not a condom

    Quinoa = Not a condom

    Breath = that's not a contraceptive mate, don't you even try it!

7. Trying to open the condom using just your energetic phallus will prove tricky, so maybe just use your hands. Once the condom is on, you may commence your union and have a lovely time. Off you go.

Marc: Sorry Fran. You're bending my penis back at a funny angle and it's a little bit painful. I'd like to stop.

I wasn't sure why exactly but I started to cry and he said (while gazing in wonder at one of my tear drops glistening on his fingertip), '*This* . . . is . . . beautiful.'

I snottily replied, 'I really thought it was going to work this time. I did EVERYTHING right. We looked into each other's eyes LOADS. We didn't touch for ages, we breathed together, you saw my aura – you said it was orange . . . which is, to be honest, a little bit disappointing, but even with all that something still went wrong. Maybe I'm just not meant to have sex.'

And he didn't try to fix it, he just lay there, stroking my hair as we fell asleep, listening to the sounds of other people having orgasms all around us through the thin tent canvas. I thought I'd made so much progress at Sex Camp. I was also impressed how easily and clearly Marc could articulate his pain and ask for the sex to stop, without worrying how I'd react. Why did I struggle so much to do that? I think I was crying because I'd put so much pressure on the experience. (I'd gone and bought a tent and witnessed it being blessed just so I could stay an extra week!) It was like trying to lose my virginity all over again, I'd made it too important. Again.

The next morning, I wanted to go home, I was completely exhausted and drained. I sat, whispering at the back of the early morning meditation class, with my friend from outside the Love Lounge.

'Don't go,' he said. 'Just stay until the end of the week.'

'Focus!' came the sharp shrill voice of the meditation workshop leader from the front of the room, causing many participants to jolt out of their deep relaxation with little shrieks. They followed the leader's gaze and scowled at us; we had clearly torn the mindful atmosphere to shreds.

'There's one workshop you could try,' my friend continued, 'I think it might really help. It's a vagina worshipping workshop. I think it might be exactly up your . . . street.'

We were told off by the workshop leader for not focusing and are advised to move to different ends of the room if we couldn't control our unbalancing behaviour.

'You probably need to sign up for it, it's always really popular . . . it would be a real shame if you left without having your vagina worshipped though.' He smiled at me and closed his eyes to avoid the gaze of the meditation teacher, who was striding towards us to separate us like kids at school.

I had taken many workshops at Sex Camp. The eight-handed massage workshop (one of the loneliest experiences of my life), Naked Ecstatic Dance class (one of the friendliest experiences of my life), Creative Body Painting (I was still getting green paint out of my pubes for weeks).

It was on my last day at Sex Camp, towel in hand at a Yoni Worshipping workshop that the most significant thing happened. I was lying down on my back, in a room of about thirty couples. Incense smoldered, windchimes underscored everything, and everyone with a vagina had a partner gazing at it and a tiny bowl of lube by their sides.

I'd nervously umm'd and ahhh'd about asking Marc to do this workshop with me. It's hard to know how to ask someone if they'd like to come and gaze at your vagina. It felt like a really big deal for me, especially from someone, who at sixteen, made her boyfriend turn out all of the lights, just in case he might get the smallest glimpse of what lay between her legs.

On the whole the camp had been very heteronormative. Men were described as the wine glasses to hold 'the smooth wine of women's pleasure' and most activities were partnered male and female. Ideas of gender also felt prohibitively rigid. I was told I should be cultivating my feminine essence by letting my hair hang loose and wearing dresses (terrible news for my dungarees). The Yoni Worshipping workshop was the only place where I saw any same-sex partnering, people with vaginas gazing at and worshiping each other's vaginas, quite awestruck by what they saw.

The workshop leader closed the doors, talked us through anatomy gently with a velvet vulva puppet and then began.

LEADER: I invite the worshipper to gaze upon Yoni. Describe what you can see.

Around me I heard voices exclaiming, 'Beautiful, pink like a shell, a garden, an orchid, a moist plum in a dewy meadow,' and Marc declared loudly and proudly, 'Yoni's made a little bubble!'

Right. Charming.

I craned my neck up and surveyed the class. All of the men in the room were crying.

LEADER: Yessss, it can be emotional, paying attention to something you may have rushed by or treated badly in the past.

Marc nodded at me tearfully. It was probably the longest time anyone has ever looked at my vagina, longer than a doctor and definitely longer than me. I thought of all the things that have been said about my vulva: the doctors telling me to go out and use it more, the teenage boys who called it a fish, a man who asked me to shave off all of my pubic hair before he would go down there, the person who said he didn't need to use a condom with me because he knew my vagina was 'safe' . . .

LEADER: Men, describe this experience, how is this for you?

A SMATTERING OF MEN'S VOICES ECHOED AROUND THE ROOM: Spiritual, connection, love, holy, beautiful, connected, love.

MARC: A REVERENTIAL HOMECOMING.

And I am thinking: WHAT??? My vagina is—

MARC: A REVERENTIAL HOMECOMING.

He says it again, just as loud, just as proud.

LEADER: Now women, tune in, listen to your Yoni, what is she saying?

I was lightly panicking at this point because I was going to have to make something up, wasn't I? My Yoni doesn't speak, my Yoni is silent, so I was going to have to make something up, something as good as A REVERENTIAL HOMECOMING. Something like Yoni says, 'Give penis a chance' or Yoni says . . . phone home or something like . . .

YONI: FRANCES

ME: Yoni?

YONI: FRANCES

ME: Yes?

YONI: THIS. IS. YONI

ME: The voice of my vagina?

YONI: My name is Yoni, call me by my true name!

ME: Just to check, are you speaking to me through my actual labia minora or majora lips?

I should say I have slightly dramatized this section for the sake of the book but I want you to know this is all completely true, this conversation did actually happen between me and my vagina (my vagina and I, sorry) and I feel very odd about it because I don't really believe that's a thing that happens, vaginas don't talk . . . but it really, genuinely did.

YONI: You want to know how to fix sex Frances?

FRAN: Yeah, so much Yoni!

YONI: You want to know how to graduate from Yoniveristy?

FRAN: I want to graduate from Yoniversity so much!

YONI: You won't like what I have to say.

FRAN: Hey that's a bit presumptuous, give it a go yeah, you've got the floor, the pelvic floor, amiright Yoni? Sorry, you talk, I'll listen and hopefully together we can work this out.

YONI: Okaaaay. Nothing more!

FRAN: Yup I'm listening, I'm not going to say anything more.

YONI: No. More. Sex. Unless it's special.

FRAN: Woah Yoni! Not exactly the empowered feminist message I was expecting. I want to be able to have sex whenever I want, however I want, so you can understand why 'no more sex unless it's special' is confusing for me, because I have it on very good authority that you are meant to be a—

YONI: A reverential homecoming, I know. It's a real responsibility to shoulder.

FRAN: Yoni, could you scroll down a bit, there must be a footnote or something, the message can't just be that.

YONI: There's no footnote. Also, please only wear cotton pants and get a Mooncup if you can't use the correct absorbency of tampon. Good luck.

The workshop leader brought the session to an end and asked for our final reflections. I was furious. Seething. So angry with my vagina.

LEADER: What did Yoni say? Would anyone like to share? Shall we start here . . .

I tried to avoid her gaze, but she is looking directly at me and Marc.

LEADER: Would you like to start?

Marc breathed in and sighed deeply, he placed one hand on his heart and sighed loudly. When he finished, he gestured to me.

LEADER: What did Yoni say?

ME: It–

LEADER: She.

ME: *She* said 'nothing more unless it's special' . . . but what does special mean?

The leader didn't reply, she just let out a long sigh.

I was at a Sex Camp and confused. I wasn't sure what I'd gained, other than a very confusing conversation with my surprisingly conservative vagina and a *sort of* boyfriend who it turned out was a social media manager, who enjoyed performance poetry and amateur wrestling (we hadn't talked much about our outside lives, as if the mere utterance of the fact we had jobs, lives and responsibilities might break the fragile magic of Sex Camp). I wanted a resolution, a nice neat answer, something I could take back into the outside world and start using straight away. A quick fix.

In a bid to try and find my happy ending, I went back to the first proper workshop I'd done, the consent workshop. This time I knew exactly what I wanted. I recognised a man who I'd chatted to in the sauna and asked him to talk with me, it's all I wanted, just talking. I didn't want to be touched at all. He told me about his family and his past relationships, I told him I just chatted with my vagina.

HIM: I have three sisters, all younger, one older brother.

ME: Surely *special* means love, right? So, I only have sex if I am in love? What if I am not in love? No sex? Or does special mean that I have to give sex lots of time? I don't always have lots of time, I'm very busy, I've barely enough time to begin and then give up on a wank while microwaving a jacket potato.

HIM: I grew up in Cardiff, great night life—

ME: And if Yoni is right, it means that *they* were right, the people who say wait for the right person, that sex is much better once you're in love, or married, or that I'm having too much sex or not enough sex, or too bland or too wild or too much sex with men who work in the arts. (I do have a lot of sex with men who work in the arts.)

HIM: Do you, um, want to come and see my bell tent?

ME: And if Yoni is right, I have to slow down and be with just myself and just my body and I have never wanted to do that.

HIM: Can we kiss?

ME: No thanks.

He put a hand on my knee and I simply moved it, nope, not there, not now. His face was visibly disappointed and he became distant and sulky. I kept talking, but he was restless, brooding and dismissive. Eventually he stood up and walked out of the room, slamming the door behind him loudly.

People's heads turned, brought abruptly out of their work-shop giggling and caressing, they then followed his flightpath with their eyes and saw me sitting alone. And I . . . well, I just sat there. I wanted to go after him and tell him that it's not him, it's me, he's lovely and I'm sure lots of people would want to kiss with him, but I personally have just had a massive chat with my vagina and just want words right now. I wanted to tell the people in the workshop peering at me curiously, hungry for what had just happened that it wasn't what it looked like, and nothing had *happened,* that I hadn't done anything wrong, that I'd just said 'no'. But I didn't.

I had for the first time in a really long while, actually been true to what I wanted and not felt like I'd had to justify myself.

Later that day as Marc and I left Sex Camp, sat on the same train, the oxytocin began to wear off.

'How are you feeling?' he asked.

'Just answering some emails, I have missed so many emails.' The minute we were in range of signal my inbox had started to fill up and I was fidgety, worrying about not having replied to people, having disappeared entirely off grid for two weeks.

'No. That is what is going on for you. How *are* you? You don't have to tell me with words, you can tell me with silence.' So, we sat there in silence, me trying to beam how I was feeling into his head. Stressed. Stressed. Stressed.

Marc asked a man who sat down opposite us if we could have the space for ourselves, it is our last time together for a while and we'd like to have it *intimately* for ourselves. I flashed the man an apologetic smile of thanks for moving, worrying he thinks we are going to have sex on the train, whereas intimacy for Marc means gazing into each other's eyes until we pull into London. In the mirror in the train toilet, I saw how wild I looked. I hadn't looked at my reflection for a while, and I looked glowing but deeply exhausted.

I wanted so much to hold onto the peace I'd found at Sex Camp. I promised myself I would live striving to be special and sensual in all things. I told myself I would always light candles to make love and never rush eating a Pret-a-Manger sandwich between meetings (I would even chew each mouthful many times before swallowing), but when a man pushed a snack trolley down the carriage, I ordered a beer and a Kinder Bueno and crammed them in my mouth without even thinking. Marc took out a large bag of seeds and ate them pointedly and mindfully one at a time.

As we left each other I got flustered at the ticket barrier with the sudden onslaught of ping ping ping ping pinging from my phone, rejection emails from work, people wanting things from me, my normal life rushing in to overtake the calm of Sex Camp. At Sex Camp I had learnt to focus on only myself and my body. I hadn't had to prove myself to anyone, or be successful, or try too hard. My normal life was nothing like this. My normal life was going to feel very hug-deficient.

Marc and I tried to keep our romance going. I visited him a few times. When I arrived, he met me at the train with a rose, had run me a long bath, lit candles and erected his massage table. When he visited me in London, he stood outside my meetings waiting for me, wanting to spend every possible moment with me strengthening our bond, he got upset if I answered my phone while we were together, bursting the bubble of our connection. We tried energetic sexting, but my energetic phallus wouldn't reach to Whitstable. Eventually he ended the relationship that we both knew only worked at Sex Camp. It felt like having a romance during a school play, falling in love while playing characters of Sandy and Danny in *Grease* but then in the real world realising that there's nothing holding your Summer Loving together.

Still, I was hopeful. Yoni had told me not to have sex unless it was special and so I tried to make intimate encounters special. I'd light incense, but dates would find it distracting and tacky. I'd ask dates if we could breathe together and look into each other's eyes, but I was told it was a mood killer. If sex seemed on the table I'd ask if we could focus on non-penetrative sex, but the response was always, 'Uh huh, foreplay, the bit before the sex, I love the bit before the sex'. I had all of these new tools, but didn't know how to use them outside of Sex Camp.

Somehow, I was further away from fixing my broken vagina than ever before. I had the knowledge that my body *could* work, *did* work, but I didn't know how to give it the things it needed among all the other demands on my time and life.

And so, I stopped trying to fix sex.

And when I stopped trying to fix sex, suddenly things did start to happen.

* * *

Vulva Massage

The idea with vulva massage isn't to have an orgasm, but to be touched intimately without the pressure to perform for a partner (or for yourself if doing it solo). The benefits can be a deep relaxation, connecting yourself with your genitals, getting used to touch and pleasure without the pressure of a goal. It is something that can be done with a partner, on your own or administered by a professional. There is no official certification for tantric yoni massage, but anyone offering it should have training in physiotherapy or a certificate in massage therapy. I'd spent some time considering booking myself in for a professional vulva massage, handing my vulva over to a pro, but at this point it wasn't something I felt safe doing. It was something I needed to explore on my own. If you are doing this with a partner, know that there is no pressure to reciprocate, this massage is about honouring yourself and allowing you space to explore.

Instructions for a vulva massage

Don't start by thinking about orgasm, take that pressure off entirely.

Have a think about the set up: maybe some music, low lighting (it's a cliché but it genuinely does help with the release of oxytocin).

Turn your phone off and get yourself into a comfortable position – cushions, throws, whatever makes you feel safe and relaxed – somewhere you aren't going to be disturbed.

Take everything really slowly, as slow as you can possibly go while still feeling connected to your body.

Spend some time settling your body and just breathing. Once you feel ready begin to run your fingers over your body, pay attention to your abdomen, your upper and inner thighs, your chest, but also just anywhere that feels good.

Use massage oil or lubricant if that feels good for you. Experiment with different pressures and speeds, use just one finger, or the palm of your hand, fingers spread or together, or your nails (gently).

When you are ready, use the palm of your palm to hold your vulva and just be still. Start to move your palm in circles, this just wakes everything up.

Gently do a few pelvic squeezes and draw your breath in deeply from your pelvic floor. If you like the sensation give the hairs on your pubic mound a gentle tug, this will bring blood flow and awareness to the area.

Run your lubricated hands from bottom to top of your vulva in long upward strokes. Work from the outside in, start with your outer lips and use your hands to sandwich them together. Experiment with pressing them together and releasing them. Then take each individual lip, gently clamp it between your thumb and forefinger and make circles up the length of the labia. Run your lubricated fingers along the gap between your inner and outer labia.

Then massage your inner lips, massage them together and then each one individually, stretch them gently, pull them gently, stroke them gently . . . I'm saying the word 'gently' a lot . . . of course experiment with pressure, but I'd say best to start gently in this highly sensitive area and build up to a pressure you like.

If you would like to touch your clitoris, use a pincer grip and massage over the clitoral shaft. You can also circle your finger around the clitoris slowly, varying pressure, gently tap your fingers on the clitoris, and roll the clitoris between your thumb and forefinger.

If you would like to, place a finger into the vagina (start by just going up to your first knuckle) and gently apply pressure imagining that your vagina is a clock, to each individual clock point. You can go further in about two inches, directly behind the clitoris . . . it may feel spongy to the touch and draw your finger gently over this area, apply different pressures.

Finish the massage by cupping your vulva again in your hand and breathing deeply.

Some of these steps might not work for you, or feel good for you at all, it might be enough to just stroke your legs or place one hand over your vulva, you might go straight for your clitoris. Whatever works for you, there's no one way to do it, there's no expectation on you, feeling safe, relaxed and slowed down is enough.

What I love about this exercise is that you don't have to worry about 'getting anywhere'. It's not about sexual satisfaction, it's bringing an awareness to a range of sensations and different types of touch, some you might like, some you'll be like 'nope, not for me'.

Spoiler alert: don't tell anyone, but because you take orgasm off the table there is more of a chance it might happen if you want it to, because you aren't aiming for it. Of course, don't *not* aim for it in the hope of it happening, because well that's sort of sneakily like aiming for it . . . but hey they're your genitals: do what you like. If it does end in orgasm then cool, but if it doesn't, well, it wasn't what you set out for anyway. This technique helped me familiarise myself with my body, which also means I can communicate what I like with a partner far more easily now, because I've done it myself in a low-pressure environment.

HONEST CONVERSATIONS ABOUT SEX
Sex is like . . . the tortoise and the hare

A: Female, Bisexual, she/her, 27
B: Male, he/him, straight, 35

A: Sexually we are a bit like the rabbit and the hare . . . sorry the tortoise and the hare.

B: I'm the tortoise. I don't feel the need to have sex very regularly, but I love, love, love the build-up. Sex for a while was something I felt anxiety about.

A: I'm the hare. I do have a really high libido, I'm like 'Let's go, let's go, let's go.' He was a bit worried that I was going to keep coming on to him and he would have to keep rejecting me, and I had to get used to him saying he isn't in the mood.

B: I did start to feel like I couldn't keep up and I was in the place where it was taking me longer to get hard and longer to come and we were both feeling frustrated.

A: I felt like a weirdo because I never saw girls on TV having a very high libido, but the reality is it goes both ways. The stereotype is guys having a huge libido, but it's not always the way.

B: I really struggled knowing it's ok to say I'm not in the mood.

A: One of the best things we did was we fed it into our role play. If he's not in the mood he'll say 'no' and make me wait and so it all becomes part of the build-up. It all feeds into our sexual fantasy.

B: It's how we find a positive in it rather than it being a combat.

A: I love that if something is not ok, he will tell me.

B: We do feedback at the end of every session, we'll say what worked and what didn't. It's genuinely one of the best things I think a couple can do is after sex is have that talk.

A: I didn't realise that some guys like it slow.

B: SLOOOOW, VERY SLOW. There is a pressure to be just like *bang bang bang* for hours on end but I feel really weird in positions when we are really far away from each other, I am an intimacy guy.

A: We went to a kink night and I felt so much safer there than I do in a normal club, because everyone there asks permission before they touch you. We had discussed our fantasies and one was having sex in front of other people. The people there were so nice running it, they said if we didn't know how to use any of the equipment to give them a shout and they would give us a tutorial.

B: They gave us a whipping tutorial.

A: We are just willing to try everything, always thinking about new positions, new toys, new lingerie, we are really wary of being complacent so we want to keep it fresh. But also, one of the things I really like doing is when we've had a really long day at work and he's exhausted and I'm exhausted, I'll be like, 'Hey, if I had the energy right now, I would give you so much head'.

B: And I'll say it back. It's really nice hearing that from your partner when your brain wants to do stuff but your body isn't allowing you.

A: We still like lazy sex too.

9

Talking About Sex Onstage
& Learning to Wank

So, this is where I am today and the truth is, I haven't got an answer, I haven't fixed sex. I was really hoping I'd have a nice big ejaculatory ending for you, because both a story and sex need a happy ending, right?

(Fran takes off her dolphin costume. Dolphins are the only other creatures who have sex for pleasure.)

But the way things traditionally end isn't going to happen for me, yet, and actually that's ok. And we don't have to end this story like everyone else. We can end it however we like, and finish in our own time and at our own pace.

Women vaginally lubricate every time they are praised. I'm just going to leave you with that thought.

(Fran holds a confetti cannon aloft above her head, it may or may not go off. Black out when it feels right.)

This is how my story used to end. At least in front of an audience. With me holding a confetti cannon warily above my head, bracing myself for the potential bang and ejaculatory splash of cascading glitter, that may or may not come, having just stepped out of an adult-size dolphin costume. The words above are the last words of my hour-long theatre comedy show, which thousands of people have come to watch in venues large and small. I had started talking about my vagina on stage.

I had been working as a comedian, a writer and a teacher, while trying to solve sex. I often wrote about my own life, but I definitely wasn't planning on writing about my vagina. This was mostly because I didn't think anyone would be interested in hearing about it. I pictured audience members wincing in embarrassment, realising that they were trapped in a small, dark, probably clammy room, with a woman wailing endlessly about her lacklustre genitals. When I imagined what that show would look like, it was me in a harsh spotlight, dressed in a black body stocking, using physical theatre, masks and waving a ribbon stick wildly as an expression of my sexual odyssey (with the spotlight occasionally turning red to symbolise my inner feminine menstrual rage). We can all picture *this* show (or perhaps have even seen this show; if you've been to the Edinburgh Fringe you have definitely seen this show), and it . . . well, I wasn't sure people would want to hear it.

I wasn't even sure I wanted to share my story. It would mean that EVERYONE would know that my sex life wasn't perfect. Would I be taken seriously as a writer again? Would I only attract Magic Penis Men from then on? Would I have to keep it secret at work? What would I tell my parents? I was finding any reason to not write a show about this very intimate thing, but more and more I kept coming back to the subject. Why don't we talk about the more difficult bits of sex? Why is there so much pretending around sex? Why is sex sometimes so hard?

Then one day during a week-long workshop on creating autobiographical theatre I was asked to think about what questions were at the heart of the work I wanted to make. On an otherwise blank double-page spread of my notebook I wrote one word. 'SEX?' I wasn't quite ready to be completely vulnerable and talk about being broken in front of these cool theatremakers, so I skirted around ideas of porn and over-sexualisation in the media. I explored sex education, fetish culture and phone sex, but I was sidestepping around the heart of the issue. Pain.

On the last day, we all had to present five to ten minutes of the project we'd been working on that week. I sat up late into the night, weaving together thoughts on sex and how interesting sex is and isn't sex everywhere – sex, sex, sex – but none of it felt true. None of it was true. So, I went back to the drawing board and came up with a new question: Why do I find sex so hard?

The workshop felt the safest place to share my story and if it didn't feel right, then I never had to speak about it again. The next day I presented a song to the tune of Silk's 'Freak Me' (Let Me Lick You Up and Down), but changing the lyrics to incorporate the reality of sex for me: 'Let me lick you up and down but first let me use this vaginal numbing gel.'

I was worried it would feel like I was publicly admitting sexual failure, but the response was warm, with many sharing their own stories and worries about sex with me. They said it was refreshing to offer a view of sex that wasn't airbrushed, one that was full of the worries and insecurities we all experience but rarely feel like we can talk about. The refrain that kept coming back was, 'keep talking about this, this is important'.

So, I did.

Firstly, I had to come up with a title for my show. Suggestions included:

How to do Sex
How to do Sex Right
Ad Libido
Morgasm
Great Sexpectations
Shag, you're it

In the end I went for Ad Libido and started working on the show very quietly. The people in the workshop had loved the idea, but that felt miles away from sharing with the general public. So, I decided to showcase fifteen minutes of it at a Battersea Arts Centre theatre scratch night for trying out new ideas. I didn't tell anyone or promote it in any way. I was planning on turning up, being completely anonymous, performing, realising that in fact, yes, I was right, the world at large did not want to hear about my vagina at all, go back to my job, vagina between my legs, never to mention it again.

'Give me a cheer if you've ever had sex?' I took the microphone in my hand and squinted at the room. I couldn't see anyone's faces, but an unsure cheer came back. People were nervous, suddenly shifting in their seats at the mention of the word 'sex', perhaps worried that there might be audience interaction. I took a deep breath: it was time to tell my story.

On the train home that night I was reading feedback forms from the audience, grinning to myself. Even the person who suggested that in future I do the whole performance with my legs in gynaecological stirrups and make my vagina talk directly to the audience, like in a Samuel Beckett play, seemed to have really enjoyed it. They had laughed warmly with my attempts to lose my virginity and felt empathy towards how clueless about sex you can be as a teenager. Some had stopped to talk to me afterwards; they'd wanted to share their own stories and thank me for speaking so openly about mine. It wasn't just me who found sex hard. I wasn't on my own.

The man sitting opposite me on the train home was talking avidly to his date until she got off at her stop. I could feel his eyes on me and the feedback forms on the table between us. He placed one hand on the top of the pages and slid them towards himself and slowly wrote a phone number in scrawled biro on top of an A4 sheet.

'This is my phone number. If you want to fix sex then I can help you out. Just give me a call. I'll fix you. Any time.'

I'd experienced a capsule version of the highs and lows of talking about sex in one evening: a warm appreciative audience and an invasive intimidating onlooker. It is not easy being someone who talks openly about sex.

When I was a comedian gigging regularly on the circuit, I would frequently be sent persistent overly familiar messages by men who had seen my work, men would wait for me after gigs and in extreme but not infrequent cases follow me home. This was before I started even talking about my vagina. The trouble with being a performer is that you have to promote your exact location frequently because you do need people to come to your shows and to buy those sweet sweet tickets so you can eat, but it also makes you very visible and vulnerable. I've had many experiences of men who have watched my show and felt like they knew me, like sitting in the dark and watching me share my story onstage had created a deeply unbreakable bond between us. It meant they felt they could approach me, and sometimes this has made me feel unsafe.

I did sometimes wish I wasn't writing about such an intimate subject, but the positives vastly outshone the more difficult moments. The show had sell-out runs, standing ovations, Q&A panels with sex experts. It's been performed in big theatres to large audiences, and once at a festival, where there were just a handful of people watching who had come in to the tent to get out of the rain while coming down off drugs. (They took some more drugs in time for me to jump out of a tent dressed as a dolphin . . . or perhaps the real drug was theatre all along?) I won Performer of the Year at The Sexual Freedom Awards. My trophy was a gold wooden handcrafted phallus (should be a vulva of course, but I guess you can't have everything . . . and the penis does have wings).

After the show, audience members would stop me to say they had had similar experiences, that they struggled with sex; some even told me that this was the first time they had realised it wasn't just them. People cried; one man went and phoned his wife directly after the show. Couples sometimes had the first open conversations they'd ever had about sex with each other on the way home. Lots of people told me that I now pop into their head while they are having sex . . . which is . . . nice?

Somehow, I had accidentally become a sex educator, I was on podcasts, the radio. I wrote articles for newspapers and magazines that my mother had even heard of. I didn't have any concrete answers for anyone but I was talking about vaginas and their pleasure and that seemed enough for the moment. Even the bad reviews ('Fails to penetrate'; two stars), seemed unimportant compared to the good ripple effects the show was having.

The end message of the show was one of anti-climax, that things can't all be tied up neatly when it comes to sex, that we are all different, so there is no one way we should be having or enjoying sex. That there is no such thing as normal sex. The show would end with a confetti cannon exploding, as previously detailed. Some nights the confetti cannon didn't go off, no matter how much I twisted it. Audience members often thought this was intentional, a clever narrative theatrical device, me struggling desperately with sweaty hands, a beautiful metaphor for helplessly groping with my own sex life and genitals. The audience liked it not going off so much that some days I actively tried to make it not go off, but, of course, on those days the confetti exploded with the gentlest of strokes. Another very apt metaphor for sex.

And that was where the story used to end, me finding pieces of confetti in every nook of my body for days after doing the show, but my life, my body and my sexual experiences have carried on.

I was talking very loudly about sex, extolling the values of open communication, of finding out what you want and prioritising your own pleasure. I was enjoying praise for speaking so candidly and warmly about something that people often don't discuss. And, of course, with all this vociferous positive polemical sex talk, I was absolutely practising what I preached in my own sex life.

Of course I was.

I definitely totally was.

I was. I really, really was.

Every. Single. Time.

Ok, in truth I wasn't at all. In my first sexual relationship after I started performing the show, I lost my grip on all of the progress I had made.

'Is everything . . . ok?' I asked. I was on a second date and could feel that something in the energy had shifted. He was closed off and didn't seem to meet my eye.

'I googled you when you went to the bathroom . . . I saw about your show . . . why didn't you tell me about your show and the . . . field you work in . . . the fact that it's about . . . you know . . . sex?'

I had told him that I was a comedian and a writer on our first date but had left it there. He hadn't asked what I wrote about, so I hadn't mentioned it. Rightly or wrongly, I had made the decision that as it's difficult to separate the subject of my work with the activity that could potentially happen at the end of a date; he didn't need to know . . . yet. We hadn't even kissed at this point.

'I do write about sex. I can find sex quite painful and I guess the show is about me trying to learn to enjoy it, it's mostly really fun and silly, there's a dolphin costume.'

'Why a dolphin costume? Do you have sex with a dolphin in the show?'

'No . . . it's because dolphins are one of the only animals who have sex for pleasure . . . and I guess I wanted to be like a dolphin, to enjoy sex as much as dolphins did, there's no dolphin sex, no.'

He seemed uncomfortable and didn't mention it again that evening. I was busy with my show, preparing for a tour and working on new projects, but we began to date.

As time went on, he saw me posting about sex online, which he hated.

'Every time we have sex, I keep thinking about your tweets . . . I saw one about pubic hair and how it's fine to have pubic hair and it makes me think that I'm not allowed an opinion on your pubic hair.'

I started to wish I was writing about something else, maybe a gripping murder mystery or a quaint period romance (but with no mention of periods of course). Perhaps in writing the show I had closed down the possibility of having a normal relationship ever again?

A few months in and I was en route to meet his family for the first time and he asked without taking his eyes off of the train window, 'Can you not tell my family what you . . . *do* . . . exactly?'

'Can I say I make comedy?'

'Yeah, of course, I'd never want you to stop talking about your writing, I'm so proud of your writing, I'm not *that* guy. But maybe if it's too hard to talk about those things without saying about the . . . sex stuff . . . then maybe just say that you are a teacher?'

I really hadn't planned on talking about the 'sex stuff' with his family. I wasn't clutching large diagrams of the clitoris to show his grandma and hadn't brought lube sachets for his dad . . . although I now wish I had. So, we sat with his family and walked on eggshells around my career. I curtailed and modified my answers, swerved frequently if things felt like they were getting too close to my work.

'So, you're a writer, what sort of thing do you write about?'

'Oh. Well. In my teaching job, I write on the board, I write out the questions for my students to answer and sometimes I write marks on their work.'

I felt like I was an embarrassment and had made myself a family-unfriendly prospect.

He would go quiet for ages.

I'd ask, 'What's on your mind?'

'I can't stop thinking about your show,' he'd reply.

I should say at this point, because it is probably vitally important, he had never come to see my show.

I ask myself now why I didn't end it immediately and remind myself to be compassionate and, again, to anyone who has found themselves in a relationship that feels unhealthy, it is absolutely not your fault: it is often very hard to end it. I didn't leave the relationship at that point because he told me so often that someone talking out loud about sex was undateable, that no one was ever going to want to be with me if I kept saying the word vagina so loudly, that he was doing something extraordinary in putting up with my work.

Any sex I had with him felt completely empty.

'Have you ever tried using a vibrator . . . during sex?' asked Laura.

I hadn't. Using a vibrator felt like a secret thing, something that should only happen behind closed doors, with loud music playing/near heavy machinery to hide the noise, not something you use with someone you want to fancy you.

'It's completely revolutionised my sex life,' she continued, 'I used to just use it when he was out, or away, or if he was on the phone and I knew he wasn't coming in the bedroom for a bit and I'd lock myself in the ensuite. Now I actually keep it charging on the bedside table, instead of at the back of my underwear drawer where he won't find it.'

'And he likes it?'

'He just reaches for it now and starts to use it on me. Honestly it just takes all the worry out of things, like when he's using his fingers I'm always thinking, "Oh his poor knuckle joints, he's going to wear them out" . . . and no one is going to come if they're worrying about knuckle joints, they are really important joints.'

I thought it was worth a go, something new for him and I to try together, something different that was just ours. I had bought sex toys in the past, but had shyly avoided conversations with the incredibly helpful staff in sex toy shops, because ridiculously I didn't want them to know I was buying a sex toy. Imagine if they knew I'd come to a sex toy vendor to buy a sex toy, rather than them thinking I'd accidentally walked in and somehow found myself surrounded by dildos and vibrators (many shaped like tiny penguins, dolphins and butterflies).

This time I asked for a lot of advice. A lot. I wasn't going to be lost in a sea of internal, external, clitoral suction, bullet vibrator, glass dildo, anal plugs, wands, toys that work in the bath, that you sit on, vibrating underwear, rabbits, massagers that slip on the end of your fingers, ones with remote controls . . . just to name a few. I asked sex toy shop owner Sam Evans about how to introduce a sex toy into partnered play and she suggested starting small, a bullet vibrator being a great starting point, but not to just whip it out in the middle of sex.

'Maybe say, "Do you fancy playing with this? I've been playing with it on my own and I really enjoy it." Tell them how fun it is, that it can make sex feel really good for both of you; maybe stay away from the word "better".'

I was nervous that he might not be into it, but she told me that a bullet vibrator isn't just for people with a clitoris, but is also fun on nipples and penises. She really recommended choosing something that your partner wouldn't feel visually compared to, so probably not a great big veiny dildo.

She reassured me that research always shows people are curious and interested. 'There are always going to be people who feel threatened no matter what you do, so just go for something you feel comfortable with.'

I felt confident and excited.

'I was wondering if we could try using this?' I said to him and slid a small bullet vibrator onto the bed. 'During sex.'

He stared at it; eyebrows raised.

'I think it might just help me relax and you might enjoy it too.'

'Right,' he said and turned away from me. He spent an awful lot of time turned away from me.

'It might be fun and if we don't like it then we never have to use it again.'

'If that's what you want.'

His words were positive but his tone and mannerisms felt wounded and dismissive.

'We don't have to; it was just a thought.' I slid it back into a drawer.

'I feel like you are saying I'm not doing a good enough job.'

'That's not it at all.'

'Then why are you replacing me?'

'It's definitely not a replacement.'

'I feel like I am never going to be enough for you, Fran. Sexually. It makes me feel like I'm not man enough for you.'

'That definitely isn't it.'

'But you use this on your own . . . that's already a massive red flag that you think I'm not sexually satisfying you . . . you wouldn't need this if you felt satisfied and now you want to use it when we are together?'

It had happened again. I had fallen into something that I was making myself smaller in (actually in all of the ways, he hated that I was slightly taller than him so I started to stand with a slouch to make him feel better). I was struggling to hold onto anything I'd learnt about sex or my body. In the past, I had stayed in these relationships too long, trying desperately to fix them from the inside, patching over the holes, scooping buck-etfuls of water out of what was clearly a sinking ship. I began to dislike my body and feel unattractive naked. I found myself avoiding certain topics of conversation just in case I upset him. I never spoke about my work.

I became less.

Onstage I felt empowered speaking to people about sex and intimacy. I liked who I was onstage, making a difference, gently and honestly talking about something difficult. I liked that I could make people laugh *and* learn about sex, while watching a fully grown woman turn into a dolphin. In his bed I felt weak and an embarrassment. He started to develop his own sexual problems and blamed them on me.

In the show I would sing:

Tell me when it's over, when your bit's complete
You pick up the pace and I sink into the sheets
My body's in the room
But my mind's no longer here
You think we're connecting but I've disappeared
I've disappeared, I've disappeared.

'When do you think you are going to stop performing your show?' The question came again and again from him. I started looking at wrapping up the strings of the tour and thinking about what I would make next, nothing autobiographical, nothing about sex, nothing upsetting. I started saying no to invitations to talk on podcasts about sex and booked in the last few dates of Ad Libido.

Sometimes things happen exactly when you need them to. Sometimes thing pop up just in time to remind you that what you are doing is ok. I had just performed the show for what I thought would be the last time. It had been a lovely show, with a loud, warm, appreciative audience and it was with a twist in my chest that I was meticulously sweeping confetti up from the floor for the last time. I didn't want to mingle in the theatre bar that evening. I wanted to be in the theatre space for as long as possible, just soaking in the last bit of my work, before starting a new chapter. A less vagina-centric chapter. Once I felt like the audience had left, I picked up my wheelie suitcase and turned out the house lights.

On the train home I opened an email from an audience member with the subject title THANK YOU.

Just . . . THANK YOU. I was silently crying throughout half of your Ad Libido performance, as I knew just how much my sorry sixteen-year-old self would've given to realise that I wasn't alone back in 2010. The NHS webpage was vague and unhelpful. The prospect of 'treatments' (scary vaginal dilators and psychosexual counselling) terrified me to the point that I thought I would just have to come to terms with the fact I'd never have a sexual relationship. Your art is so vital in amplifying the conversation around painful sex, around underrepresented conditions and the sheer *volume of people affected by it. Thank you for creating a platform where I can lament about the time my boyfriend berated me for 'wasting condoms' because 'they're expensive' (before you say — the free ones we got from college were a brand he didn't like) every time he tried to put his penis inside me and I just couldn't. I can only hope this reaches anyone and everyone who needs to hear it to know they're not the only ones! Thank you for being so honest and for saying it in such a fun, accessible way, all without denying that sometimes . . . sex is just really fucking hard. I hope it makes a huge difference, I hope it makes people get help and makes people do more research, but even if it's just a tiny difference, just to people on their own, who've felt scared and ashamed and broken . . . if it makes them a little more chatty, confident and comforted, then that really is enough.**

The reason I share this isn't for a little self-boost (although it really did boost me a lot and we all need a boost now and then), but because I went directly home and ended that relationship. I decided to carry on touring the show and I kept talking about vaginas and haven't stopped.

Where did that leave my sex life? Well.

After performing my show one evening a woman approached me confidently in the theatre bar.

'I've got some thoughts about your show!'

I smiled politely, hoping she wasn't a reviewer.

'You need to talk more about masturbation, it's the only thing that's missing. Masturbation is very important, talk more about it. Learning to touch myself honestly changed my life. I wish I'd discovered it earlier. Otherwise it's a great show. More

---

* Shared here with permission.

masturbation please,' and with that she turned around and exited the room.

Well, she wasn't wrong. There was one thing I had been really neglecting, both from my show and from my life. Myself.

When I asked people for their sex advice there was one theme that came up over and over again.

Engage in self-pleasure as much as you can to find out what you like. 40, f

I wish I'd have got to know my own body better when I was younger and have bought the right 'tools' to be able to do the job alone! 50 f

Masturbate, masturbate, masturbate 22, f

Masturbation, self-pleasuring, wanking: it was impossible to ignore. A tsunami of people thought that *giving yourself a hand* was at the heart of a healthy sex life.

I am not very good at talking about masturbation. For someone who talks about sex and her vagina a lot, solo sex is my Achilles clit. I get embarrassed, flustered, I try to move on to the next topic of conversation as fast as I can. Telling you about the fluff that accumulates in and around my vulva on a day-to-day basis? Not a problem. Self-pleasure . . . well, I, um . . . TAXI PLEASE! Talking about wanking makes me shy.

At school, boys bragged endlessly about how often they *tugged themselves off* (loads, endlessly, at every opportunity allegedly) and there was talk of a game called *soggy biscuit*. But there were no snack-based wanking games if you had a vulva. Any girl suspected of masturbating was immediately branded a witch and burnt at the stake . . . or the playground equivalent, which was endless cries of 'fish fingers', causing everyone else (putting their hands clearly in the air, away from their genitals) to vehemently deny that they'd ever touched themselves.

As I became sexually active, masturbation was something I associated with being single. A lonely compensation activity only to be done while reading tear-drenched letters from an ex-boyfriend, eating Häagen-Dazs ice cream and crying to Celine Dion's 'My Heart Will Go On'. If you had a partner then why would you need to touch yourself? Surely that was their job? And any self-fiddling was the equivalent of making them redundant.

How comfortable we feel touching ourselves can depend on many factors. Many people who took my survey spoke about feeling like they'd done something wrong, dirty or sinful.

It feels exposing (I have to hide under the bedcovers in order to feel safe enough to get turned on), there's just a lot of ingrained shame that I'm having to work through. Sometimes it's easy to 'get over', sometimes I have to do a bit of mental gymnastics in order to get anywhere. 21, f

I remember first experiencing pleasure when I was 4 when I rubbed myself with blankets, but I thought it was wrong so I didn't want anyone to find out. 32, f

I feel dirty when I do it and I don't like talking about it or doing it in front of my partner. I think me viewing sex and pleasure as dirty caused my vaginismus. I'm trying to become more confident at pleasuring myself in front of my partner. 22, f

217

In my twenties masturbation changed again: it was no longer a dirty punchline to a bad joke. Magazines encouraged people to explore themselves, rabbit vibrators bunny-hopped into bedside drawers and slowly, slowly in my world, masturbation was becoming associated with independence, empowerment and self-care. The message was clear: You don't need to be reliant on a partner to have a good time, keep on eating that Häagen-Dazs and wank to Celine Dion long into the night. Or day. Or whenever you feel stressed, sexy, bored, hungry, down, happy . . . any time you fancy really.

But I just wasn't.

I wasn't masturbating. Not regularly. Not really at all.

I felt like it was something I *should* be doing, something to check that everything was working, but I would get bored, distracted and still really thought it wasn't 'my job'. My pleasure had been for someone else for so long, that the thought of giving it to myself . . . well, I couldn't get my head round it.

After developing and performing my show, I was welcomed into the incredibly supportive vagina community and continuously surrounded by sex-positive messages. I had a social media timeline full of people saying that masturbation is a feminist act of freedom, a political statement, a message of independence, something I *should* be doing, two fingers up (your vagina) to the patriarchy. By not masturbating frequently and diligently was I the patriarchy?

I had felt like I wasn't getting sex right, and I now felt I wasn't getting masturbation right either, but the messages from people I spoke to were overwhelming.

Thank god for masturbation.

It was like a lightbulb coming on like 'oh! that's why people do this!!'

My masturbation record is 19 orgasms in a row aged 16. I was aiming for 20 in a night but I started feeling really faint.

Masturbation literally saved my life. Thank God for the clitoris.

Discovering masturbation in my early 20s was totally life-changing.

It was clear the thing I was avoiding and handing over to my partners, could change matters.

Laura and I were sat in her garden. We speak fairly openly about sex these days and I feel so lucky to have friends I can talk to about all things vagina. She is delighted to tell me that her thrush is under control, the doctor had been very non-judgemental and told her she didn't need to keep apologising to her personally for it. We had met that evening to check in, because in a moment of self-empowered 'sisters are doing it for themselves' glee, we had signed ourselves up for a masturbation challenge.

I'm sure I don't need to tell you that May is (obviously) the international month of masturbation, and we were planning to 'wank every day for May'. We'd heard that if we do it every day, it will increase our sexual appetite, sensation will be improved, we'll sleep better, be less stressed, period cramps might be eased and, temporarily, our immune system might be strengthened.

We have signed up together so we can make each other accountable, sending each other little 'REMEMBER TO WANK' text alerts in the evenings, to which we respond with multiple thumbs up and the occasional vegetable emoji. However, it is May the fourth, International Star Wars Day, and I have already been rubbish at going Hans Solo.

ME: I just wanted to sleep.

LAURA: Masturbation will help you sleep.

ME: I had a lot on my mind.

LAURA: Masturbation would help clear your mind and unwind.

ME: I'll catch up by doing it twice today . . . but I do have a deadline to hit.

LAURA: The more you put in the more you get out.

(Laura is now my absolute vaginal cheerleader.)

ME: All I can think is, 'Let's get this done so you can go to sleep' or 'I really should be getting on with clearing my inbox' and 'this is never going to work.'

LAURA: Did you set the scene and make things feel nice, calm and relaxed?

ME: I put an audiobook on?

LAURA: A sexy audiobook?

ME: *The Handmaid's Tale*?

LAURA: Not a sexy audiobook. You know nothing bad will happen to you if you do, right?

ME: I know masturbation will not cause me to go blind.

LAURA: Nor will any kittens die and no hair will grow on the palm of your hands.

ME: I just can't get in the right headspace.

I had a lot of blocks to overcome: making time, feeling safe, quieting the voices in my head telling me I had other stuff I should be doing, rather than prioritising myself.

To begin with I kept beating myself up if touching myself didn't feel like I expected it to (I was expecting fireworks, waterfalls and a shooting stars) or if it went absolutely nowhere. I gave myself permission to take my time, remove any goal and begin to unwind a very busy brain. The more I was patient and kind to my body the easier this became. Distraction massively reduces our ability to feel sexual sensation, so I slowed down and took the pressure off.[37] Sometimes sleep was exactly what I needed, sometimes stroking my breasts was perfect for that day, sometimes experimenting with a toy was exactly what I fancied. I tried different things from day to day, but the more I could get rid of unhelpful thoughts about the kind of experience I *should* be having, the more I found out what I liked.

I can safely say that getting to know my own body through masturbation and using sex toys has been the single best thing I have done for my sexual wellbeing. Full stop. No questions. It has in time also greatly improved my partnered sex life. In the past I might have felt that this was a crutch or an insult to my partner (surely my lover's genitals should be able to get me there on their own) but the better sex feels, the more I enjoy it, the more often I want it, the happier everyone is. Women who masturbate report higher levels of sexual satisfaction than those who don't.[38] It still makes me shy, but I'm getting better at talking about it and doing it all the time.

I'm still learning how to masturbate. There are books on technique, instructional manuals abound, there's the app

OMGYes where you can use the screen of your smartphone to learn and practice the different strokes on a virtual vulva. I read magazine articles about how to use your very clean power shower to make you very very dirty and googled multiple agony aunt Q&A's asking worriedly 'for a friend' whether or not using a vibrator could wear out my clitoris entirely . . . but really all I had to do was take my time and explore. I spoke to people, I asked the questions I was too scared to ask as a teenager, I texted Dormitory Witch lots, I even attended a squirting workshop. But also, I kept reminding myself there was no pressure. I felt like a failure for so long, for not masturbating enough. There are so many benefits to it, but anytime we set a standard or a bar we are adding an unnecessary pressure and pressure isn't sexy. We should be in touch with our bodies . . . when and if we feel like it and if we lose interest half way through or we've had enough then that is also fine too. There is so much pressure in life already, our bodies are trying so hard to be good bodies all the time, so let yourself shed any expectations, throw out those *should's* and just take it easy.

Treat your body with kindness, celebrate where it is today and remember to be curious . . . take the hard and fast rules out of it . . . unless hard and fast does it for you, in which case, go for it.

I would love to present a manual here of ways to get in the mood and different masturbation techniques but every vulva is different. Everyone's life experience is different. Everyone has different fantasies and different things that get them going. It would be really ridiculous for me, someone who really just started on this journey to give instructions or direction. What I'd like to do is share a few of the survey answers, in the hope of showing a range of experiences, some that might feel familiar, some that feel far away from your own personal experience, in the hope of sharing the fact that, whether you've been masturbating for years or days, whatever you do you are completely and utterly normal.

How do you masturbate?

Take your time. Stop thinking. Start feeling and listening to the body. We're often encouraged to rush into chasing orgasm. But including every part of the body, and taking time to move at a pace that is comfortable makes it much more satisfying. 39, f

If you own a clit and a shower head enjoy that partnership. Also don't wank for the sake of wanking – it's so much better if you are actually horny. 28

Give yourself time and space to do it, no interruptions, or worries your housemates/family might hear what you're up to. The fewer inhibitions the better. Then get yourself comfy (sofa, floor, bath, bed – wherever feels good) and start exploring your body – start by stroking yourself all over your body and see what feels nice, you might be surprised what turns you on! You don't have to go straight for your genitals, or touch them at all! Take everything at the pace that feels good to you and your body will tell you what it wants! 33, f

Faster and harder does not necessarily mean better. Your ideas of yourself and what you like may be something you've formed over time that doesn't feel true anymore. 22, f

Lots of lubrication and some dirty thoughts. And make sure the cats are out of the room. 44, f

BUY A VIBRATOR!!! Or several. 23, f

Ignore whatever you think everyone else does and find what works for you for a shame- and guilt-free experience. For example, I find vibrators (switched on) desensitising and ultimately disappointing but clearly other women don't. I prefer to use them switched off rather than my own fingers. Don't worry if it's all about the clit and nothing about the vagina. I was concerned about this for years, pointlessly. 46, f

I like to keep my pants on and never put anything inside myself. 22, f

Take your time, don't go straight for gold, touching around the clit and helping everything to fire up really helps with the intensity. Don't forget to breathe. 35

* * *

Body Positivity

Sexy Selfie

The internet is flooded with articles and guides to taking a sexy selfie or nude for your lover, but for some people taking photographs of themself *for* themselves can be an important part of self-love. The more positive and comfortable we feel in our bodies, the more enjoyable sex is.

Start by practising self-care on your body, whatever that means for you, have a luxurious bath, moisturise, exercise, dance, masturbate, eat a massive pie, dress up, dress down, whatever you do treat yourself really good. Put on some music and arrange yourself a place where you will feel safe and relaxed. There is no pressure on this, so take time to play with lighting, get creative with your Anglepoise lamp, light some tea lights, lie in bed with the sunshine pouring in your window, bask in the electric light of your computer screen. You can either set a timer or use selfie mode, but experiment with taking photographs of your body at its most sensual, whatever that means to you.

To begin with I really struggled with this task. I wanted it to be something empowering and full of self-love and self-acceptance. What I found instead was I was looking at these images critically. My body didn't match up to what I thought it would look like in my head, none of the pictures were 'good enough', they showed folds and stretch marks and bits I'd learnt to dislike. I tried not to pose, I tried not to do faces that felt copied from porn. I tried to capture myself at my most *myself*, but I kept on focusing on my flaws.

I got quite upset by it and so left it that day. Sometimes it's equally important to know when something isn't quite right for you. I realised I had been taking sexy selfies as if they were going to be sent to a lover, or seen through someone else's eyes. I was still taking them for other people and not for myself. I was worrying about what the recipient would think upon receiving them, but the recipient was me. When I started to look with celebratory eyes, I began to see the joy, movement and vitality of my body and stopped looking at myself as an object for other people to place worth on.

Life Drawing

Studies show that attending life drawing classes has a positive effect on body image, and that participants can increase their body image satisfaction from the beginning of a class to after class and be 25% happier at the end of a class.[39] So . . .

1. Attend a life drawing session as an artist (it really doesn't matter if you think you can't draw, and it doesn't matter if you make the model's fingers look like bananas, fingers are hard to draw). In a class you will look at a range of bodies, which are all incredible, different and wonderful. In drawing you'll begin to celebrate the human body; see all the amazing things it can do!

2. Have a go at being a life drawing model. Now this may seem like a big jump from attending a life drawing class as an artist, but it's been one of the most liberating things I've ever done. I'm not suggesting you sign up as a professional life model and tour art schools; I've heard experiences from life model friends that those spaces don't always feel safe. I went to a body-positive life drawing event, *Body Love Sketch Club*, where everyone draws and anyone who wants to be drawn can pose. It was amazing to be drawn just exactly as I am, draw other people in return and realise the kindness and attention with which we were appreciating other people's bodies and know that we can be that kind with our own. If you can't attend a lovely safe workshop like *Body Love Sketch Club*, then construct your own. Draw your body in the mirror or from a photograph. I did one with a friend, stripping off and drawing each other

over Skype. Lying there being drawn I felt like an absolute goddess (as per usual a bit worried someone might walk in and wonder why I'm laying naked in front of my laptop) but I found myself looking at my own body compassionately and actually with a lot of love when someone else was looking at it in an artistic way. I felt like a work of art.

HONEST CONVERSATIONS ABOUT SEX
Sex is surplus to requirements

Genderfluid, asexual biromantic, pronouns any, 30

If I had known about asexuality when I was younger, I wonder how differently things would have gone for me.

The word 'asexual' came up for me about five years ago now. I'd always struggled with sex and I'm an actor so I got very good at performing sex enthusiastically because I loved the people I was in relationships with. I definitely had a romantic connection with them and for me at that time this went hand in hand with having sex and so, I thought, 'I am broken and I will keep working at this until I am not broken anymore'.

I'd been seeing the doctor about this and they said, 'You just need more lube, go home and use more lube'. I did, and then came back and said, 'We have used LOTS of lube, we are sliding around on the bed and it's *still* not happening'. I was given a topical general anaesthetic to put in my vagina to stop the pain, but being completely numb and trying to have sex at the same time was an utterly bizarre experience. I had one session with a sex therapist; she gave me homework and when I got back home I realised that even if I could make all the sensations feel right, I still wouldn't have any desire to actually have sex and it was a little while after that when I found asexuality.

I found the word 'asexual' on a random web forum and I thought, 'This is me; this is who I am.' It was scary at the time, there was that 'AHA' moment of going, 'I'm not a broken person, *this* is exactly who I am', but also, 'I'm in a relationship with someone I love and how does this now work if this is who I am, what happens now?' I had romantic desire, but the sex side of stuff there was just nothing going on there for me; it was surplus to requirement.

228

I'm still in a relationship, my partner is allosexual. I'd say we still have sex. I think people have different fixed ideas of what sex means, a lot of people say sex is penis in vagina, penetration, getting to orgasm, and everything else is not as good as that. We've expanded our definition of what sex is . . . are we naked together? Are we in bed? Are we touching each other in ways that are pleasurable? That is sex for us.

It's not a lacking. It is so important to say it is not a lacking. A lot of people when they hear about asexuality go, 'Oh that's awful, you are missing out on something so wonderful'. For people who are asexual and aromantic, they reach satisfaction at a different level and that's ok, their life is just as full. The only thing that really causes distress is that feeling of not fitting in and not being able to see yourself represented anywhere. I remember talking to my mum about this, I was expecting her to be like, 'That's ok, this is a thing that you'll work through and you'll find ways that you can deal with it', but for her she was like, 'This is really important, sex is really important part of life' and I think a lot of people get the message, 'you're broken, you are missing out'.

I've had people who've been trying to chat me up – I don't say I'm in a relationship, I say 'I'm sorry, I'm asexual' – and I've had people say, 'Oh what a waste'. One of the big things to deal with is people who are worried about the fact that you are ok with being asexual, because in their mind if they didn't want to have sex that would be a medical issue. Asexuality was only declassified as a mental disorder in 2013, up until that point if you went to your doctor and said I'm not interested in having sex, they would say 'you are broken and we shall fix you' and even now their first port of call is that it's a hormonal imbalance or Hypoactive Sexual Desire Disorder.

I know if a doctor had mentioned asexuality to me, that would have changed the route that I would have gone on much earlier.

10

The Happy Ending & The Beginning

This book ends with me astride someone in bed.

We had been writing hotly erotically charged letters to each other for months, describing in detail what we would like to do to each other. We are both writers, so the use of metaphor, meter and alliteration is really next-level literature. There have been artistic nudes, incredibly well lit, with each photograph subtly pushing the sexy envelope . . . who knew you could be titillated by the suggestion of the shadow of a pube just out of frame? Turns out you can. I have spent this time as a single person, trying to work out what I like, learning mindfulness, my anatomy, taking long baths, relaxing, self-touch. I try learning not how to make my body work, but how to work with my body. I am trying to not see myself as 'broken' or 'a bit hit and miss sexually' or 'not wired up right', I concentrate on the positives. The positives are that I feel desire in me for the first time in a long time, I'm looking forward to being physically intimate with someone and I feel confident that I will be able to be honest with them.

We have both had to be really patient, both looking forwards to the point when we will get to be in the same room for long enough to have sex. And because we have been so beautifully patient, we deserve lovely sex. Sex that is as kind and compassionate as we have been over this period of time waiting. Sex that mirrors the tenderness that we have built up between us. Who am I kidding? Explosively pleasurable sex, because we've really done the ground work and deserve something lovely in return.

After all of that build-up, all that time trying to get to know my body . . . sex was painful. I felt more broken than I had in a very long time, because I thought I'd worked out an angle, and an amount of lube and a set of moves that worked for me and my body, but there I was again back at square one.

We started to talk.

I told him that it had been painful. I took a long breath, and another and then a few more, because well, breathing is important.

We continued talking.

We spoke about what we like and the things we were worried about. We drew our own enthusiastic boundaries, told each other how much we fancy each other often and our conversation was full of small touches, gentle pressures. He told me stories of his own, things that helped me understand how to touch him and removed any sexual landmines from the bed, so neither of us were going to accidentally step on them mid-sex.

We kept talking.

We walked to the sofa, got out a massage oil and we started again. We shared things we were curious about trying and placed gentle 'nos' on the things we thought we really wouldn't like, dropping in a few tentative 'maybes' because through talking we were creating a safe space for ourselves, for the sex we would like to have. We began from the start, unlearning the things we'd learnt elsewhere and thanking each other when we let the other know that something wasn't working. It wasn't always easy or straight forward, but the consent was loudly present and joyful: questions, nods, words, directions. We were playful and inquisitive, making suggestions without the fear of getting it wrong.

We keep talking.

When it doesn't work, we have our moments of emotion. I allow myself a small sulk, but then put music on and dance, because it gets us out of our brains and into our bodies and mostly it brings us back to sex . . . but sometimes we just dance. Dancing *is* a lot like sex. We laugh a lot in bed. We do a breathing exercise that a couple I interviewed recommended to me and we feel like complete wankers, but actually have to admit there is *something* in it. Turns out breathing is very, very important.

I realise now that this is what my vagina meant, when it told me: No more sex unless it's special. Special doesn't have to mean love, or that you are in a committed relationship or even that you have to light a single tealight. It means only having sex when you *really* want to have sex and only with people who you feel comfortable and safe with. People who will understand if you say 'no' or 'I'd like to try this' or 'how about we do it this way?' which I know sounds incredibly basic, but I so often neglect those things.

I would love this book to end with me, sitting happily, independently masturbating on a golden beach as the sun sets in front of me, enjoying sex every single time I choose to have it, loving every inch of my body enthusiastically, and feeling completely confident about speaking about sex. I hope I am on my way.

Our sex lives for the most part aren't linear. We are always learning, changing our minds, our tastes. Our bodies develop (when I started writing this book my ears used to yield incredible results, but now they are just so–so . . . my toes on the other hand have arrived at the party), hormones fluctuate, relationships open and close and our idea of what sex is isn't stationary. For every moment I feel primally connected with the great big yoniverse in the deep forest of my own sexuality, there are times of feeling totally unsexual or angry at my body for not being 'juicy' enough. What I try to be is kind to myself and not let the labels I use in those moments stick.

So, this is my happy ending.

Except for it isn't really an ending. It really is just the start. If I ever start using the word broken for my vagina or body, I remind myself:

That lubricant is brilliant!

That sometimes someone won't have an erection or be wet 'enough' but it bears no reflection to what is going on in their head.

That you can ask for someone to slow down, speed up, try something different, or stop at any time.

That communication is at the heart of good sex and that means listening as well as talking.

That sex can be gloriously messy, so sleep with people you enjoy being messy with (even if that just means yourself).

That what works with one partner, may not work with someone else, so throw out the rulebook and just ask, ask each time, ask again. Keep asking.

That if a doctor dismisses you then you can ask for a second opinion and that there are places to go for help, support and community.

That there definitely isn't anywhere near enough support for sexual difficulties, not by a long way, but hopefully things are beginning to get better.

That you can do whatever you like with your pubes.

That faking your enjoyment of sex doesn't help anyone. Nothing can get better until you start being honest about how everything feels.

That it is ok to say no at any time, even if it is a one night stand, or you are deeply in love with them or are married to them or if it's an expensive special occasion, even if they've booked a hotel, even if it's your wedding night, even if there are eight of you involved in a sexual tryst and you've all had to arrange childcare to be there, any time, ANY TIME.

And that ejaculation doesn't equal the end of sex.

And that virginity is a social construct, you 'lose' nothing when you first have sex.

And that you can leave at any point.

And that you are not untrusting if you ask them to wear a condom.

That if they take the condom off during sex that is a crime, it's called stealthing.

That semen is not a low-carb option no matter how much they say it is.

That you don't have to have sex, you can just hug, or eat or watch a film.

That if you want to have sex, you deserve safe sex.

If you want to have sex, you deserve good sex.

If you want to have sex, you deserve the best sex.

HONEST CONVERSATIONS ABOUT SEX
Sex is a playground

Female, bisexual, she/her, 26

I escort, but it's a very different type of sex. It is for *their* pleasure rather than mine and they've never made me orgasm from sex, I just don't allow it. I hold my orgasms back for my partner. With my boyfriend there is no performance, but with escorting it is all a performance, a show: lights, camera, action. I don't want to fake it with my boyfriend, so I'm really honest if something isn't working with him. My boyfriend is up for starting to escort. We are quite modern, I guess. It's something I enjoy, I'm not ashamed of it.

I have a personal relationship with sex and a work relationship with sex. It never feels like work when I have sex with my boyfriend because it's doing what I want to do. A client can say, 'Oh I want to do role play' and I'll reply, 'I love role play', but it's not my fantasy, it's theirs. I think it's really important for working girls to have partners because before my boyfriend the only sex I was having was work, so sex became so much more about the other person and sometimes . . . I want to be selfish.

Sex is a playground, explore it and have fun.

Epilogue

Dear 16-Year-Old Me

I'm sure sex will get better. Things are always hard at first but get easier with time. Right? I bet it won't be long before I'm having AMAZING sex, every single time.

– Diary of Teenage Fran

I wonder if 16-year-old Fran had known what I know now, what her sex life would have looked like, and where mine would be now as a result. I wish I could tell teenage Fran that by her early thirties she had completely fixed sex, but I haven't. I wish I could give her the tools to stop her silently disappearing in bed for all those years. I wish she could know that even though she feels like she is on her own, she isn't.

There is still a really long way to go, but it feels like there are so many more open conversations happening now than the ones she was having in 2003. 16-year-olds now talk so much more confidently about sexual fluidity, and how romantic and sexual attraction isn't just one rigid box that you have to cram yourself into. There are websites and forums dedicated to learning about and feeling safe in your body and sexuality. I wish all this had been available to her.

Imagine if I could sit her down, draw her some enormous diagrams and tell her that she isn't broken at all. What would that conversation be like?

16-YEAR-OLD ME: Woah, woah, woah, that's it?! You didn't fix sex? This is the big ending? Bit of an anti-climax!

ME: 16-year-old me! It is so good to speak to you! No, I didn't fix sex, not completely. I do know lots more about my own body though and my brain and-

16-YEAR-OLD ME: Not completely?? Great! Wonderful. Well thanks so much, so glad to have all that to look forward to, I think I'll commit myself to a life of abstinence right now. CREAK! That is the noise of my vagina shutting up shop! Shutters down. Closed for business, while everyone else is having groundbreaking sex!

ME: They really *really* aren't. Most people are still just working it out, no matter how long they've been having sex for. You are going to hear so many negative messages about sex over the years, about how your body doesn't look right, smell right, feel right, do the right things-

16-YEAR-OLD ME: Oh god, do I turn into one of those feminists who burns their bras?

ME: Yeah, you actually do, but being a feminist is great . . . although you will never burn a bra. They are really expensive and your boobs change size all the time so when you find one that actually fits, you will really stick with it . . . sorry, sidetracked . . . Where was I?

16-YEAR-OLD ME: Feeling that my body doesn't *smell* right?

ME: Your body smells fine! It smells wonderful actually. And your vagina definitely doesn't need to smell like a spring breeze or ocean spray anyway. In fact, all of your body is just glorious and so deserving of all of the good things in life. I want to protect you from so much! I want to steer you away from the unhealthy relationships you will get into and defend you from the damage they will do. I want to stand in your corner, a weird sort of sex hype woman and fill you with the confidence to be able to say 'No' or 'Yes' and truly completely mean it and-

16-YEAR-OLD ME: This is all a bit Ghost of Sex-mas Yet to Come for me. Haha . . . come.

ME: It's quite hard talking to your 16-year-old self about sex you know. I could draw you a diagram instead?

16-YEAR-OLD ME: It's ok, I won't interrupt.

ME: No, it's good actually! Keep talking, keep interrupting, keep asking questions. I want your voice to take up space. At the heart of really good sex is communication, so talk to your partners. The expectations on people with penises are huge. They are meant to *always* want sex, always have rock-hard erections and be able to last for hours and hours in bed, but this simply isn't realistic, so take some of the pressure off for everyone. Talk.

16-YEAR-OLD ME: I will let them know! DEAR ALL FUTURE LOVERS, I WILL BE TALKING TO YOU A LOT—

ME: Great, but also don't worry about *them* so much, it's so much more important to learn what *you* like and to feel comfortable asking for it.

16-YEAR-OLD ME: But I don't know what I like . . .

ME: Yeah, you're going to have to spend some time working that out. On your own. You have a pretty good working knowledge of the penis, right?

16-YEAR-OLD ME: Yup . . . the shaft, testicles, head, frenulum—

ME: Which is mad because you haven't got a penis! You do however have a vulva! You don't know anything about the clitoris or the crura or the vestibular bulbs or that the clitoris gets engorged when you're aroused just like a penis does . . . but you can name the frenu-lum?! Go and get your hand mirror, have a proper look.

16-YEAR-OLD ME: Maybe later. I'm quite stressed and busy right now, I have A levels and working out if I still fancy Ant and/or Dec. To be honest, I feel anxious quite a lot of the time.

ME: I think you are doing great. You do suffer from quite a high level of anxiety though. The part of your brain that day to day keeps you safe needs to shut down enough to really enjoy sex, so the more you can immerse yourself in places you feel relaxed and look after your mental health the better.

16-YEAR-OLD ME: Mmm, the year is 2003, mental health education might actually be even worse than sex education, but I will try to take it easy. Is there anything else?

ME: Start tracking your periods. You'll have weeks
where you'll firmly believe that you are the worst
human in the world and deserving of only unkind
and bad things . . . but you are not the worst, you are
just premenstrual. And get off *that* contraceptive
pill . . . there is more than one type of pill and *that*
one is not right for your body at all, do some research
and talk to a doctor about what might be right for
you . . . that particular one will make you cry for days
and when you come off it you will feel more yourself
than you ever thought possible. It's also fine to use
condoms.

16-YEAR-OLD ME: But what about *their* sensation? I
heard that wearing a condom means you can't properly . . . connect?

ME: You'll connect just fine. Find something that *you*
are happy with.

16-YEAR-OLD ME: Ok, well, I feel like I am totally
ready now. Bring on the sex.

ME: The most important thing is, if you don't want to
have sex with them, don't have sex with them. Don't
worry about their feelings or reaction to this. Don't
just do it to be polite, or kind, or because they feel
sad, or to check if they still fancy you. Also, the man
with his hand in your back pocket is stealing your flip
phone, not fondling your arse.

16-YEAR-OLD ME: Look, all I really need to know is
will I ever have sex like that scene in *Titanic?* You
know the scene I mean . . .

ME: I'm sorry to say that so far, you haven't made a
steamy handprint inside a condensation-covered

carriage, with either Leonardo DiCaprio *or* Kate
Winslet, but I'll keep trying. I can promise that you
will have the most intimate, silly, sensual fun enjoying
and exploring your body.

16-YEAR-OLD ME: So, I'm not broken?

ME: No, you are not broken at all.

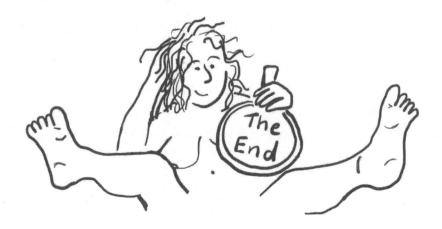

Notes

1 https://www.weforum.org/agenda/2018/04/women-are-still-not-asking -for-pay-rises-here-s-why/#_ednref2

2 D.A. Frederick, H.K.S. John, J.R. Garcia, *et al.* 'Differences in Orgasm Frequency Among Gay, Lesbian, Bisexual, and Heterosexual Men and Women in a U.S. National Sample'. *Arch Sex Behav* 47, 273–88 (2018). https://doi.org/10.1007/s10508-017-0939-z

3 *The Science of Orgasm.* Barry R. Komisaruk, Carlos Beyer-Flores, Beverly Whipple. The John Hopkins University Press. 46.

4 https://sexualadviceassociation.co.uk/womens-sexual-problems/

5 https://www.acog.org/womens-health/faqs/when-sex-is-painful

6 http://news.bbc.co.uk/1/hi/health/4111360.stm

7 *Sexual Behavior in the Human Female.* Alfred Charles Kinsey,.Institute for Sex Research, Wardell B. Pomeroy. 352.

8 Pujols Y, Seal BN, Meston CM. The association between sexual satisfaction and body image in women [published correction appears in J Sex Med. 2010 Jun;7(6):2295]. *J Sex Med.* 2010;7(2 Pt 2):905-916. doi:10.1111 /j.1743-6109.2009.01604.x

9 *Better Sex Through Mindfulness: How Women Can Cultivate Desire.* Lori Brotto. Greystone Books

10 Ibid.

11 Ibid.

12 Ibid.

13 https://eveappeal.org.uk/news-awareness/know-your-body/

14 *Better Sex Through Mindfulness: How Women Can Cultivate Desire.* Lori Brotto. Greystone Books

15 Val Wongsomboon, Mary H. Burleson & Gregory D. Webster (2020). 'Women's Orgasm and Sexual Satisfaction in Committed Sex and Casual Sex: Relationship Between Sociosexuality and Sexual Outcomes in Different Sexual Contexts', *The Journal of Sex Research*, 57:3, 285–95

16 Kennair, L. E. O., Wyckoff, J. P., Asao, K., Buss, D. M., & Bendixen, M.

(2018). Why do women regret casual sex more than men do? *Personality and Individual Differences, 127,* 61-67.

17 Wongsomboon, et al. 'Women's Orgasm and Sexual Satisfaction in Committed Sex and Casual Sex.

18 Come as You Are: The Surprising New Science That Will Transform Your Sex Life. Emily Nagoski, Blackwell's

19 https://www.nhs.uk/pregnancy/labour-and-birth/what-happens/episiotomy-and-perineal-tears/

20 https://www.theguardian.com/society/2019/jan/21/cervical-cancer-smear-test-rate-plummets-survey-young-women-smearforsmear-campaign

21 https://www.theatlantic.com/health/archive/2018/04/j-marion-sims/558248/

22 https://www.thepharmaletter.com/article/viagra-sales-to-reach-1-billion-in-first-year

23 Ray Moynihan (2003). 'The Making of a Disease: Female Sexual Dysfunction', BMJ, 4 January; 326(7379): 45–7. DOI: 10.1136/bmj.326.7379.45

24 Ibid.

25 *Law and the Regulation of Medicines.* Emily Jackson. Hart Publishing, 2012, 136.

26 Josefson D. FDA approves device for female sexual dysfunction. *BMJ.* 2000;320(7247):1427.

27 Baid R, Agarwal R. Flibanserin: A controversial drug for female hypoactive sexual desire disorder. *Ind Psychiatry J.* 2018;27(1):154-157. doi:10.4103/ipj.ipj_20_16

28 https://www.bmj.com/bmj/section-pdf/778631?path=/bmj/349/7980/Feature.full.pdf, *BMJ* 2014;349:g6246

29 https://www.thecut.com/2016/09/how-addyi-the-female-viagra-won-fda-approval.html

30 https://www.thehastingscenter.org/the-score-is-even/

31 https://www.independent.co.uk/news/people/gwyneth-paltrow-goop-jade-eggs-vaginas-gynaecologist-doctor-jen-gunter-a7541301.html

32 Brewer G, Hendrie CA. Evidence to suggest that copulatory vocalizations in women are not a reflexive consequence of orgasm. Arch Sex Behav. 2011 Jun;40(3):559-64. doi: 10.1007/s10508-010-9632-1. Epub 2010 May 18. PMID: 20480220.

33 Frederick, et al. 'Differences in Orgasm Frequency Among Gay, Lesbian, Bisexual, and Heterosexual Men and Women in a U.S. National Sample'.

34 K.S. Fugl-Meyer, K. Oberg, P.O. Lundberg, B. Lewin and A.A. Fugl-Meyer (2006), 'On Orgasm, Sexual Techniques, and Erotic Perceptions in 18–74-year-old Swedish Women', *Journal of Sexual Medicine,* 3, 56.

35 https://www.omgyes.com/en/members/pairing

36 https://bettymartin.org/the-bossy-massage/

37 A.B. Anderson and L.D. Hamilton (2015), 'Assessment of Distraction from Erotic Stimuli by Nonerotic Interference, *Journal of Sex Research,* 52:3, 317–26.

38 A.A. Carvalheira and IP Leal (2012), 'Masturbation among Women: Associated Factors and Sexual Response in a Portuguese Community Sample', *Journal of Sex & Marital Therapy,* 39, 347–67.

39 https://aru.ac.uk/news/life-drawing-classes-have-positive-effect-on-body-image#:~:text=%E2%80%9CThese%20studies%20indicate%20 that%20life,depictions%20of%20'idealised'%20bodies.

Resources & Further Reading

Some wonderful books

Come As You Are, Emily Nagoski

Vagina: A re-education, Lynn Enright

Better Sex Through Mindfulness: How Women Can Cultivate Desire, Lori A. Brotto

Doing It: Let's Talk About Sex, Hannah Witton

Vagina: A New Biography, Naomi Wolf

The Vagina Bible: The vulva and the vagina – separating the myth from the medicine, Dr. Jennifer Gunter

Women on Top of the World, Lucy-Anne Holmes

Me and My Menopausal Vagina: Living with Vaginal Atrophy, Jane Lewis

Private Parts: Living well with bad periods and endometriosis, Eleanor Thom

Mind The Gap: The truth about desire and how to futureproof your sex life, Dr Karen Gurney

Queer Sex: A Trans and Non-Binary Guide to Intimacy, Pleasure and Relationships, Juno Roche

This Book is Gay, Juno Dawson

For more information on possible causes of painful sex

thevaginismusnetwork.com

vulvalpainsociety.org

eveappeal.org.uk

endometriosis-uk.org

For sex education

Brook.org.uk

sexpression.org.uk

decolonisingcontraception.com

For registered sexual and relationship therapists

COSRT.ORG.UK

For erotica

tabitharayne.com

For lubricant

yesyesyes.org

For sex toys

JoDivine.com (shop and advice)

Sexwithashley.com (sex toy reviews)

For support with abusive relationships

relate.org.uk

womensaid.org.uk

nationaldahelpline.org.uk

For mental health

mind.org.uk

For LGBTQIA+

asexuality.org

Stonewall.org.uk

There are so many incredible sex educators and activists on social media to follow and learn from. Fill your timelines with important, educational and kind content, look away from your screen every twenty minutes, be gentle with your brain and stay hydrated.

Acknowledgements

I imagined writing a book would be a very solitary, *lock yourself away in an attic and only emerge (as a husk) when the last full stop is placed* activity. It is a bit like that (I am definitely a bit husky), but this book is also a big lively celebration of so many people and so much talking. *My Broken Vagina* would never have got down on the page without the kindness of people who really believed in it and me. Big thanks to everyone who kept me writing it, I am beyond lucky to have had your support.

To everyone at JULA, you really are the friendliest agency. Huge thanks especially to Rachel Mann for believing I could write a book, having only seen me transform into a dolphin onstage. I feel so proud to be represented by you and look forwards to writing many more books!

Thank you to everyone at Hodder Studio. I can't wait to meet you all in person and see more than just your heads and shoulders on zoom calls. Big thanks to my editor Myfanwy Moore, for being so smart, gentle and perceptive with my story, to Izzy Everington, for kindly steering this newbie through the world of books and to Jo Myler for the perfect cover design and trying so many different caterpillars. To Ellie Wheeldon, Callie Robertson, Dominic Gribbin, Veronique Norton, thank you for helping my book get out into the world and finding creative ways to say 'vagina', 'orgasm' and 'sex' in a world that sends emails containing those words straight to the spam folder.

A huge thank you to the vagina community. You are the most welcoming of communities. If I ever write a book about my nasal passage, I can only pray that the nose community will be as warm. Big thanks to Sam Evans, Lavinia Winch, Tabitha Rayne and The Vag Network. To the people who gave up their time to speak to me about their sex lives, thank you for generously sharing your most personal of stories. Thank you to everyone who took the time to fill in the sex surveys, even the bots . . . I am very glad I could provide a safe space for bots to share their sex worries.

To ALL of the Laura's in my life. Thank you for all the advice, support and pep talks along the way. Thanks to Amelie Roch for going above and beyond; I am going to take you to Decorate a Dildo to say thank you the minute we are allowed out. Big kisses to Lisa Mackenzie, we might never have met if we hadn't both had 'broken' vaginas. To every friend who has replied to my 'Does the world really want to hear about my vagina?' texts late at night with affirmative 'Yes, yes they really do'. To everyone who was patient when I had my head stuck far too far up my own vagina, I love you lots and will take you for a pint to say thank you soon. To James Rowland for bringing me plates of food in the shape of different smiley faces and reminding me to ask for help when I needed it. I really am terrible at asking for help, but people were always overbrimming with ideas, love and support.

To everyone who has supported me with my writing, helped me work out how to speak about my vagina, sung about my work from the rooftops and poured a large glass of wine when needed: Ellen Havard, Annie May Fletcher, Laura Horton, everyone in the workshop run by Briony Kimmings, Sarah Blanc, everyone at The Pleasance, Kate and Andy at Shiny Button, Hilly Fletcher, Katie Langridge, Kate Turner, Emma Harpley, Perdita Stott, Ashleigh Laurence, Lucy Atkinson, Amala Anyika, Daisy Hale & Sean Brooks. Thank you for having my back.

Thank you to my parents, for having my winged penis trophy on your mantelpiece, my show posters on your walls, and always being very proud and supportive. Also for all the cake.

I wrote this book during a time when we weren't allowed to properly see or touch each other. So, to everyone that made that a little easier, thank you from the very bottom of my vag.